ADVANCE PRAISE FOR *LEAN MOM, FIT FAMILY*

"This important book is the first to address the nutrition and fitness needs of the entire family. Michael Sena and his coauthors place emphasis on lifestyle change where it needs to be—in the family as a whole, instead of the individual."

—Charlotte (Toby) Tate, Ph.D., former president of the American College of Sports Medicine and dean of the College of Applied Health Sciences at the University of Illinois at Chicago

"Wow! Finally a book I can recommend to families that understands fitness is a family affair. Not only is the advice sound, but the concept of working together is bang on!"

—Cathryn Tobin, M.D., pediatrician and author of *The Parent's Problem Solver*

"Michael Sena is a passionate advocate for healthy families, and it comes across loud and clear in his book. Moms who open this book will be pleasantly surprised to find that Michael has given them simple and reasonable tools to get the job done—including sample agendas for family meetings, easy-to-follow menus, and age-specific activity recommendations for children."

—Matt Longjohn, M.D., M.P.H., executive director of the Consortium to Lower Obesity in Chicago Children

"Michael Sena has done an outstanding job educating communities (in Chicago) that healthy lifestyles are not about the sacrifices you give up but about, more importantly, the benefits that you reap! Taking simple steps to incorporate smart eating, more activity, and a better life just became easier!"

—Colleen Lammel-Harmon, R.D., L.D.N., senior program fitness specialist, cochair of the Mayor's Fitness Council—Chicago Park District

"*Lean Mom, Fit Family* is the perfect plan for moms who want to shape up, slim down, and enlist their families' help and support. Michael Sena's enthusiasm guarantees that moms will get excited, stay motivated, and be unstoppable as they work their way through his 6-week plan."

—Cynthia Kersey, author of *Unstoppable* and *Unstoppable Women*

"Michael Sena's practical and hands-on suggestions are perfect for moms who don't have a lot of time to get fit, and his upbeat attitude is sure to inspire readers toward success."

—Lesley Marcus, Kids Café coordinator at the Greater Chicago Food Depository

"In *Lean Mom, Fit Family*, Michael Sena and his colleagues offer clear, practical step-by-step advice you can use to improve your own weight and health—and that of your whole family! Michael has it just right, with his emphasis on health for all members of the household. Take it from a father of five—family power is a key ingredient in lasting improvements to fitness, nutrition, health, and weight. I commend this book to you. It is full of the rarest, common thing I know: abundant good sense!"

—David L. Katz, M.D., M.P.H., F.A.C.P.M., F.A.C.P, Yale University School of Medicine

The **6**-Week Plan
for a Slimmer You and a Healthier Family

Lean Mom, Fit Family

MICHAEL SENA, C.F.S.

with Kirsten Straughan, R.D., L.D., and Tom Sattler, Ed.D.

RODALE

Exercise and stretching photographs by Mitch Mandel / Rodale Images. All other interior photographs by Julie Fabifzak.

Book design by Tara Long

Library of Congress Cataloging-in-Publication Data

Sena, Michael.
    Lean mom, fit family : the 6-week plan for a slimmer you and a healthier family / Michael Sena, with Kirsten Straughan and Tom Sattler.
        p.   cm.
    Includes index.
    ISBN-13 978–1–59486–067–6 paperback
    ISBN-10 1–59486–067–X paperback
    1. Family—Health and hygiene. 2. Mothers—Health and hygiene. 3. Physical fitness. 4. Reducing diets. 5. Weight loss. 6. Nutrition. I. Straughan, Kirsten. II. Sattler, Thomas P. III. Title.
RA777.7.S46 2005
613.2'5—dc22
                                                     2005008769

Distributed to the trade by Holtzbrinck Publishers

2 4 6 8 10 9 7 5 3 1   paperback

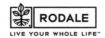

To my mother, Francesca, who jump-started my fitness career
back when I was 3 years old by putting me in front of the television
to watch The Jack La Lanne Show.

To my father, Cesario, who always told me, "If you're a Sena, you can't fail."

And to my first college weight-room buddy, David Guiliano Jr.,
who taught me how to lift weights and exercise the "right way."

Contents

Foreword

By John Hefferon, M.D.

As a practicing orthopedic surgeon for 25 years, I have witnessed our nation's increasing focus on physical fitness.

Around 1975, the running craze took hold, and the sight of people running along roads and sidewalks was no longer considered to be unusual. Sports medicine emerged, as the general population wanted to be treated like the premier athletes they watched on television. A new industry based on running shoes and sports apparel became part of the nation's economy. Exercise physiology and nutrition became everyday topics of household conversation. Words such as *aerobic* and *anaerobic, concentric* and *eccentric exercise,* and *delts* and *abs* have come into general use. The popularity of long-distance running has created a strong interest in marathons and triathlons. Those who eschew running have become involved in other activities such as aerobics, step aerobics, kickboxing, and Spinning.

Americans are privy to a mass of information on diet choices for increasing muscle mass, losing weight, and controlling cholesterol. Some of our previous diet platitudes have come into question as research has unearthed new information about relative values of various food groups. All of this has occurred in a population that's increasingly on the go and susceptible to the lure of fast food.

Despite the wealth of information available about healthy lifestyles, people continue to search for a program that works consistently—a program that will help promote fitness, be compatible with their busy lifestyles, and be applicable to future generations.

Michael Sena and his collaborators, Kirsten Straughan and Thomas Sattler, have put together a family fitness plan that can work for the American family. It is based on sound principles of nutrition and exercise physiology and can be used by any age group.

Why is this book so invaluable?

The authors are recognized experts in fitness and health, with decades of experience. Michael Sena's reputation as a personal trainer is unparalleled. His techniques are strongly based on scientific knowledge and avoid gimmicks and fads. He is cochairman of Chicago Mayor Richard Daley's Fitness Council and is seen all over the world as the fitness expert for United Airlines. Despite his worldwide reputation, Michael continues to work as a personal trainer on a daily basis with his loyal clients. He is constantly in touch with the practicalities of health and fitness.

Kirsten Straughan, mother of two, marathoner, and dietitian, has had a lifetime interest in family fitness. Her years of experience in sports nutrition, metabolic education, and family counseling make her uniquely qualified in her field. This book benefits greatly from her practical insights into family nutrition.

Dr. Tom Sattler's 40 years of experience in teaching exercise physiology components at the university level as well as supervising professional athletes' physical training give him a unique perspective on fitness at all training levels. He currently trains exercise physiologists in the Senior FITness division of Alliance Rehab, a Health Resources Alliance company. Dr. Sattler knows the importance of developing a lifetime fitness plan.

Any family fitness plan must have a built-in flexibility to accommodate individuals without straying from the basic concepts. This book provides such a program.

The plan must have "legs." It must be designed to last a lifetime. Lifestyles and preferences change with time. Developing a lifelong fitness program starts with this 6-week program, yet this book goes beyond that, helping to teach healthy habits that will benefit your family for years to come.

On a final note, I encourage you to use this book to expand your horizons on fitness and nutrition. Let this publication pique your intellectual curiosity. Become familiar with the terminology so that you can appreciate new concepts in this ever-changing field of science. Use this knowledge to improve your family's health and happiness.

Dr. Hefferon is an orthopedic consultant to the NBA, the impartial examiner for the NFL, and president of both the Medical Association of Chicago and the Chicago Orthopedic Foundation. He was the team physician for the 1996 Olympic basketball team and the six-time world champion Chicago Bulls.

Acknowledgments

When my editor told me that the only thing left to write for this book was the acknowledgments, two things came to mind. First, I knew we were really finished—finished like college was finally over. Second, I could now thank the long list of individuals who helped me write this lifelong dream and much-needed book, and who deserve as much credit as I do in their own special way. Individuals don't write great books; gangs of people do. Here's my gang!

So many thanks and consideration have to go to my business partner and good friend, Arthur Ashley, for without him, this book certainly would never have happened. Arthur has believed in me for many years, and when it came time to financially support me, he was the only one left standing. To my associate and nutritionist, Kirsten Straughan, who worked countless hours on this book while maintaining her practice; giving birth to her second child, Sofie; and taking care of her 5-year-old son, Jack, and her husband, Anton. And did I mention that she also sold her home and moved into a new one? She is the true definition of a Super Mom, and her input will be so valuable to every mother who reads this book. To my college professor, surrogate father, brilliant teacher, and an all-around great human being, Dr. Tom Sattler. I have learned so much about physiology—and more important, about life— through you. You are and always will be a driving force, and I can't thank you enough for being by my side. To Dr. John Hefferon, one of the country's foremost and most respected authorities in the field of orthopedics, who graced me with the honor of writing the foreword to this book. Dr. Hefferon has worked with professional athletes from all sports, most notably

Michael Jordan, and he has been instrumental in helping so many of my clients (and me too) get back on our feet and continue to do the things we love to do. Thank you.

To my assistant Mark Paulson, who has typed every word that I have written in this book—thank you for connecting me to the 21st century! To Lou Cinquino from Rodale, who believed in this project more than any other publisher. I can't thank you enough for giving me my start in the world of book writing; I will make you proud. To my editor, Amy Super, who at times had me in fits of rage over her revisions and corrections. Because of you, I now know what a well-written book is supposed to look like. Thank you for your professionalism and determination in molding this book to be the great work that it has become. To my book designer, Tara Long, who has put together a layout and "look" that even the perfectionist that I am can only marvel at. You do nice work. To Bill Reishtein, my brander and literary agent, who put this deal together. Thank you always for your hard work and endless drive.

Everyone should have an Uncle Louie, as I have. He is truly one of the most inspirational and knowledgeable men that I know and has always provided me with the wind for my sails. Uncle Louie, you always taught me that I can't do everything alone and to surround myself with good people—thanks for being one of them! To my first family of fitness here in Chicago, the Smolins. Eddie, Susan, Matthew, and Sammy—thanks for the start, the meals, and most important, the love. To my lifelong New York buddy and friend, Ron Kramer. Thank you for all of your nutritional guidance over the years. Your knowledge is head and shoulders above the rest, and the time has come for the world to recognize that. I would also like to thank my business associates and sponsors who have opened doors of opportunity for me that would not be possible if it weren't for each and every one of you: Spri products, Lifefitness, United Airlines, Pace Communications, Marriott Hotels, WGN-9 TV in Chicago, WMAQ/NBC-5 in Chicago, Mayor Daley's Fitness Council, CLOCC, and Kid's Café.

I would like to mention a special thanks to all of my personal training clients who have supported me and my dreams. You've allowed me to cancel appointments during this past year so that I could finish writing this book, but that doesn't give you a hall pass to skip your cardio! To my former business partner, Jenny Lorbeck, whose love and support have afforded me the time to write this book, and who has taught me about the "gentler" side of life. I will love you always. To Larry Potash, one of the country's best news anchormen (even though you are from Boston and cheer for the Red Sox), I am indebted to you eternally for helping me get my start on television. Your integrity is as solid as a rock—"Go Yankees!" To Paul Konrad, the funniest weatherman on television today, you have taught me many things: the art of an effective "tease," how to talk to a television camera, and most important, how to look inside myself and find out who I really am. For that I thank you and love you.

Finally, I must thank one of the greatest inspirations in my life today. When I first met Chazz Palminteri, we were both doormen at the Limelight nightclub in New York City. Chazz was, yes, the struggling actor. Little did I know that someday he would be one of Hollywood's most talented and respected artists. To me, Chazz is the poster child for perseverance and has been a great friend and consultant to me in all areas of life. Thank you for all that you and your wife, my friend Giana, have done for me. Most of all, thank you for the love and inspiration!

Introduction

This is a book for you, and most of all, for your family. My hope is that it will allow you to give your family a precious and priceless gift—a lifetime of health and fitness. I've spent my entire adult life working to help all types of people feel better, both physically and emotionally. After 24 years as a personal trainer, I know how badly people want to make improvements and how much of a struggle it can be. I've always dreamed of writing a book that would show just how easy—and rewarding—it can be to live a healthy lifestyle. I also knew that if I could share the success stories of inspiring people I've met, I could help others achieve the same kind of dramatic results.

But it wasn't until I put together a story for my regular fitness segment on a Chicago morning news program on NBC Channel 5 that I knew I had to write *this* book. On TV early one Wednesday morning, I expressed my concern about the "overweight, underfit" status of today's adults and, sadly, today's children. I announced that I was going to work with one family in Chicago for 6 weeks to help them transform the health and fitness of their entire family. I invited families to contact me and tell me why they should be that one family.

I have to admit, I expected maybe 30 to 40 responses and a relatively simple selection process. My segment aired at 6:00 A.M., and I thought most people would be sound asleep. Wrong! Instead, my e-mail system crashed when hundreds of messages came pouring in within the next hour—and several hundred more letters showed up on my desk over the next several days. This idea of a family approaching health and fitness together had struck a chord with the viewing audience. After reading all the heartfelt stories of families who were reaching out for help, I finally chose the Cuebas family and then gave millions of TV viewers a chance to witness their family fitness progress for 6 weeks—the good and the bad.

The Cuebas family's story really touched me. Janet Cuebas, mom of the family, was 50 pounds overweight and was worried because her family had a history of diabetes. Victor Cuebas had just lost his job and with it his health insurance, so he was also very concerned with keeping the family healthy. Their two children were average weight, but they knew that their family was not eating right. They actually sat their mom down one day and pleaded with her to prepare healthier meals! Making matters more complicated, Janet had been diagnosed with depression and was taking medication to control it.

It's easy to see in this family, as in so many others, how things can snowball into complex and difficult situations. The Cuebas family needed something to help them get on a healthier track. Once they started my 6-week program, the family dynamic began to change very quickly. Janet really took the nutrition to heart, and she started revamping the family meals. Brown rice replaced white. Her heavy use of cooking oils changed to lighter use of healthier oils, such as olive oil. High-fat meats were replaced with leaner protein sources, such as skinless chicken breasts. Janet, along with the rest of her family, started to exercise regularly.

BEFORE YOU START

Before you get started on your 6-week plan, you'll need to get medical clearance from your family physician for everyone in the family.

Your family physician is part of your fitness plan. Get your doctor involved from the start, since he will be an important part of your support system. Make sure that each physician who cares for your family is informed of what you are undertaking, and have each provide you with exercise and nutritional medical clearances for your family members. When it comes to a support system, the more, the better!

While it took a few weeks for the Cuebas family to really get on track, they reached their weight-loss and fitness goals—and then blew right past them. They were back on television 6 weeks later, and they were happy, healthy, smiling, and absolutely delighted with the way they looked and felt. Best of all, they were excited about the positive new lifestyles they had adopted. As I was writing this section (about a year after I met the Cuebas family), I called Janet to check in. She had lost 50 pounds and kept it off. Her husband had lost about 20 pounds and kept it off too. The kids were more active than ever, playing lots of soccer, and the family was very happy and enjoying each day. Best of all, Janet found that her new healthy lifestyle helped regulate her depression, and she's now off her medication!

I wrote this book because I know that you and your family can experience the same wonderful results. It disappoints me to see people unhappy about the state of their health, resigned to always feeling that way. It bothers me even more when parents pass this mind-set on to their children. It's time to pass on something more positive.

This book will help you achieve your fitness and weight-loss goals. Just give me 6 weeks in your home, and you'll see the kind of wonderful results that I know you want for yourself and for your family!

PART 1

The Seven Principles of Family Fitness

I am very excited for you and your family and for all of the positive changes that are about to enter your lives. For me, one of the most rewarding things in life is getting the opportunity to help improve someone else's health. I never get tired of seeing the expressions on people's faces when they tell me that they feel great about having finally shed unwanted pounds and about how they have become truly involved in fitness. I get even more pumped when an entire family reports to me that their health and wellness have dramatically improved. For me, this is success. There is nothing sweeter in life than having *the wealth of good health*!

I know you are going to succeed. First and foremost, you will succeed because of the commitment you will make to yourself and your family. I'm confident that you possess the drive and mental fortitude that it takes to get your family on a healthy track. The fact that you are reading this book right now tells me that you are serious about taking control of your family's health and fitness. I will be your family fitness coach. I bring more than 20 years of education, practice, and experience to you through the pages of this book. I'm going to guide you—step by step—through a program that works. I'm here to help you incorporate a no-nonsense program into your family's daily lives (along with a few healthy shortcuts) to ensure that you achieve your desired results.

The premise of my plan is very simple—and that's why it works. I'm going to provide you with Seven Principles of Family Fitness. Then, I'm going to give you a 6-week program that gets you in the habit of incorporating these principles into your life and into the lives of each member of your family. I have learned through hundreds of clients that when family members support each other and embark on a fitness program together, they succeed. That's why the focus of the book is your family.

Mom, it starts with you. You're my coach in your home. You're going to experience the difference in the way you look and feel. I promise you, if you follow my program, you will lose unwanted pounds. Six weeks from today, you will have more energy and vitality. You will be in better overall health. You will be on the road to a lifetime of healthy living!

Once you and your family have committed to doing what is necessary to improve your health, the next step is simply a matter of incorporating my seven basic principles of exercise and nutrition into your life as a family.

Just think about it: seven simple food and lifestyle changes that will create weight loss that lasts a lifetime. As thousands of my clients can attest—it works. Let's get to it!

MICHAEL SENA'S SEVEN PRINCIPLES of Family Fitness

Principle 1: Get moving!

Principle 2: Manage portion sizes

Principle 3: Eat optimum amounts of protein

Principle 4: Add fiber and switch to complex carbohydrates

Principle 5: Choose the right fats

Principle 6: Calories still count

Principle 7: You are what you drink

PRINCIPLE 1

Get Moving!

"Get moving!" Every speaking engagement, every TV appearance, and every personal training session that I do includes these two words. I hope that if I say it enough, people will really take it to heart and begin to energize their lives. You can make it your family's mantra too. Over the past couple of decades, Americans by the millions have stopped moving. This is especially true of our kids, whose computers, video games, cartoons, cell phones, and pagers have taken the place of backyard dodgeball and running around the neighborhood.

It's not enough just to eat healthy foods. You must also participate in regular physical activities. One cannot be done without the other; they are both vital components of a successful fitness program. At times, my clients try to do one without the other—but it always shows up in their progress reports. Whenever the weight isn't coming off, they admit that they either slowed down on their activity or ate too many foods that were high in saturated fat or refined sugars.

Without activity, what happens to your body is not pretty—the musculoskeletal structure that you had when you were young ages right before your eyes. Movement keeps your heart, your muscles, your bones, and your joints functioning at optimum levels. That's why you and your family need to make movement and activity part of your daily lives.

Can you give me 20 minutes of activity per day? Or should I say, "Can you give *you* 20 minutes per day?" Feeling good is a gift you can give to yourself—and it all begins with my favorite two words: *get moving.*

This may require a shift in the way you approach each day. You have to start by adopting a proper attitude about being active. Fitness will be part of your daily life, like making the coffee, brushing your teeth, or picking up the morning newspaper. You will look in every nook and cranny of your day for opportunities to squeeze in activity, because you know how good it will make you feel. I urge you to try this new attitude on for size. Throughout this book, you'll find dozens and dozens of suggestions for incorporating activity into your daily patterns. Hopefully, you'll then make your move—literally.

As we create your family's activity program together, I'm going to show you how to channel your efforts into four fundamental types of exercise. By following the plan and combining these four types of exercise, you will lose weight and gain health.

Cardiovascular exercise. Vigorous aerobic activity is essential for a healthy heart and healthy lungs. Like any other muscles in your body, your heart and lungs get stronger with use. Activities such as walking, biking, running, and swimming require your heart and lungs to work harder to support the effort. Have you ever heard the term "muscle atrophy"? This is a condition in which unused muscles wither away. Don't let this happen to your heart and lungs. In Week 1, I'll show you how to keep them pumping!

Lean muscle building. As calorie-burning tissue, muscle is the enemy of fat. The more muscle you have, the more energy (calories) it requires to stay alive. Best of all, muscle burns calories both when you are exerting yourself and when you are not—even when you're sleeping! When you exert your muscles, they go searching for energy sources, and one way they get energy is by gobbling up fat cells.

SENA SAYS:
Activity increases the body's metabolic rate to help it become a calorie-burning furnace!

Strength training is a double whammy against fat: You burn calories through the actual exercise, and your muscles burn calories as they increase in density. You don't have to be a professional bodybuilder to benefit from strength training. In Week 2, I'll show everyone in your family how to build healthy, lean muscle.

Core strengthening. Expand your thinking beyond "great-looking abs." Svelte abs will come as a result of healthy eating habits and exercising your abdominal muscles, oblique muscles, and the lumbar region of your core. By strengthening these three muscle groups, you will also help protect your spinal structure and strengthen your lower back. Core strengthening can reduce back pain as well as give you the firm, toned waistline that you have always wanted. In Week 3, I will show you a host of exercises that will strengthen your core.

Flexibility and stretching. Remaining flexible reduces your chance of injury, and it also keeps you from losing your range of motion as you get older. You want your muscles, tendons, and ligaments to be resilient, not tight and brittle. This will make all of your activities easier and more enjoyable. In Week 4, I will show you how to stretch all of your muscle groups to keep you limber and graceful.

Each of the first 4 weeks of my 6-week program will show you and your family how to focus on one of the four fundamental areas of exercise. In the last 2 weeks, I'll show you ways to integrate each of the exercise types into your weekly fitness plan. In addition, I'll provide you with weekly fun family activities that get you all moving together.

Remaining active is the key to a healthy lifestyle—and a vibrant, happy, dynamic, and positive life. This book will help you get your family moving in a very healthy direction!

PRINCIPLE 2

Manage Portion Sizes

The supersizing of nearly everything we eat has supersized our waistlines! Over the past 3 decades, the number of overweight children has nearly tripled, and the number of overweight adults has quadrupled.

Since it is clear that food marketers are not going to control portion sizes, it's up to you. Controlling portion size is a key element in bringing your body to a state of controlled and manageable weight. It's as simple as this: In order to lose weight, you must burn more calories than you consume. And since you're probably the one with the most influence over the food your family eats, it's up to you to help them understand how much to eat.

Think of your body like your car. You fill the car with gas, drive down the highway, and burn up the fuel. However, if you leave your car sitting still and go back the next day and pump in more gas, eventually the tank is going to overflow. Well, it's the same with your body. If you keep ingesting calories without activity, you'll see the "overflow" on your hips, buttocks, waistline, and thighs. When you start revving up your activity level, you can begin to eat more without having an unhealthy overflow.

PORTION SIZE CAN MAKE A HUGE DIFFERENCE IN YOUR WEIGHT

Remember, the restaurant industry has not made it easy on us when it comes to determining an appropriate portion size. I'm sure you have seen gigantic piles of pasta and enormous mounds of french fries when eating out. Although we as adults may remember a time when the portions were more reasonable, our kids certainly don't.

A recent study by the Centers for Disease Control and Prevention has found that over the past 30 years, our calorie intake has increased by 200 to 300 calories a day—which can easily occur from eating larger amounts. In practical terms, this translates into an extra 25 pounds a year. Now look at this situation in another way: If you ate 250 fewer calories every day by eating smaller portions of food, you could lose that same 25 pounds in 1 year!

The excessive portion sizes in America are even more apparent when we compare the serving sizes in fast-food restaurant chains in Europe with those here in the United States. A recent study found that the "extra large" soda at McDonald's in Dublin, Rome, and London are the same as the "large" size in America. And the "large" french fries in the United Kingdom contained 446 calories, while the "large" in America contained a whopping 610 calories!

You can remedy this situation—for yourself and for your whole family.

MICHAEL SENA'S TIPS for Reducing Portion Sizes

- ❏ Dish up portions in the kitchen or immediately put leftovers in the fridge; you'll be less likely to go back for seconds.
- ❏ Avoid eating in front of the TV or computer or while standing up. Pay attention to your food and enjoy it.
- ❏ Don't buy large quantities of "trigger" foods—those foods that you have difficulty resisting. If you have a desire for cookies, buy a single-serving package instead of a whole box.
- ❏ Share an entrée with a friend or family member when you go to a restaurant.
- ❏ Ask for half of your meal to be packed for you, then eat it for lunch the next day.
- ❏ If there's a food that you really enjoy that shouldn't be a routine part of your meal plan, occasionally order the smallest size or split it with a friend.
- ❏ Eat from a smaller plate. Visually, it will seem as if you're eating more.

GUIDELINES FOR PORTION SIZES

The following charts are intended to help you become more aware of reasonable portion sizes. For example, many of us may be used to eating mounds of pasta when, in fact, ½ cup is equal to one serving. If this doesn't sound like a lot of food, consider that a tossed salad with 1 tablespoon of dressing and 1 cup of fat-free milk can round off your pasta dinner quite nicely. Also, the number of servings you eat will depend on your weight goals. To help you, I've included weekly meal plans in part 2, with portion sizes customized to your weight-loss goals.

When looking at the following portion sizes, compare them with what you are currently eating. Do you tend to eat a whole bowl of nuts while watching TV? Or ¼ pound of cheese at a sitting? Do you tend to dump on the salad dressing until your lettuce is soggy? If your current portions are larger, it could be a major reason that you've struggled with weight loss.

PORTION SIZES FOR TEENAGERS AND ADULTS

FOOD	PORTION SIZE	VISUAL CUE
Bagel	1 small	Hockey puck
Beans	½ cup	Rounded handful
Bread	1 slice	2 CD cases
Butter or margarine	1 tsp	Your fingertip
Cheese	1 oz	Your thumb or 2 dominoes
Chocolate	1 oz	Pack of dental floss
Chopped raw vegetables	1 cup	Baseball
Dry cereal	¾–1 cup	Tennis ball
Fish	3 oz	Checkbook
Mayonnaise	1 Tbsp	Your thumb tip or lipstick cap
Meat and poultry	3 oz	Deck of cards
Milk	8 oz	1 cup

FOOD	PORTION SIZE	VISUAL CUE
Nuts	1 oz	2 full shot glasses
Pasta	½ cup	Rounded handful
Peanut butter	1 Tbsp	Your thumb tip or lipstick cap
Plain yogurt	8 oz	1 cup
Potato	1 small	Computer mouse
Raisins, dried apricots	¼ cup	Golf ball or large egg
Rice	⅓ cup	Custard cup
Salad dressing	1 Tbsp	Your thumb tip or lipstick cap

PORTION SIZES FOR CHILDREN

When discussing children's eating habits, I don't get too concerned about the amount of food kids are eating. I feel that the *types* of foods they're eating are far more important for their health and weight. However, for some general guidelines, see the chart below. It is good to have an idea of the amounts that kids of a certain age should be eating to ensure that they are getting a good balance of the nutrients they need.

FOOD	PORTION SIZE BY AGE		
	1–3 years	4–6 years	7–12 years
Bread	½ slice	1 slice	1 slice
Cereal	¼ cup	½ cup	¾ cup
Cheese	¾ oz	1 oz	1 oz
Meat and poultry	1–2 oz	1–2 oz	2–3 oz
Milk or plain yogurt	½–¾ cup	¾ cup	¾–1 cup
Pasta, beans	¼ cup	½ cup	½ cup
Vegetables and fruits	2–4 Tbsp	¼–½ cup	½–¾ cup

PRINCIPLE 3

Eat Optimum Amounts of Protein

As anyone who dines with me knows, the center of my plate is always filled with a serving of lean protein. I also recommend that my clients emphasize protein in their meal plans, but most important, I stress the importance of *lean* protein. For your program, I'm going to suggest higher protein levels than you may be accustomed to eating. These guidelines are based on the positive results I have seen in my own clients, along with recent research that touts the benefits of a higher-protein diet. A meal plan high in protein has a long list of benefits. Protein-rich foods . . .

❏ Speed up your metabolism and promote an increase in lean muscle mass, causing your body to become more efficient at burning calories, even at rest.

❏ Reduce sugar cravings. The number one question I hear from clients wanting to lose weight is "How can I stop these sugar cravings?" Sugar cravings can be caused by blood sugar fluctuations, and the best way to stabilize your blood sugar is to decrease the carbohydrates in your meal plan (particularly the simple carbohydrates) and increase the lean protein.

❏ Slow your digestion, making you feel full longer. High-protein foods slow the movement of food from the stomach to the intestine, which results in a prolonged feeling of satiety.

❏ Reduce your risk of heart disease, stroke, diabetes, hypertension, and obesity. The

Nurses' Health Study, an ongoing study of more than 100,000 women, found that over a 14-year period, women who ate the most protein were 25 percent less likely to have heart attacks or die of heart disease than women who ate the least amount of protein.

Health issues such as cardiovascular disease and diabetes are no longer of concern just to adults. The high rates of childhood obesity are resulting in serious health problems. I commend you for taking the first step toward teaching your children healthy lifestyle and eating habits!

HIGH-PROTEIN DOES NOT MEAN HIGH-FAT!

Many diet books recommend a higher-protein diet, but they unfortunately also promote protein-rich foods that are high in saturated fat—at the expense of your health. Basing a diet on foods high in cholesterol and saturated fat works against everything you want to achieve—a healthy heart and a healthy weight.

Instead of eating loads of bacon and fatty beef, try to shift your food choices toward lean animal products, such as skinless and white-meat poultry, lean beef and pork, eggs, and low-fat dairy products. But remember, there are also plenty of vegetable-based protein sources, including legumes, beans, and vegetarian soy options such as veggie burgers and veggie hot dogs. These vegetable-based proteins provide additional health benefits due to their high fiber and phytonutrient content. To make this transition as easy as possible for your family, I have outlined many options for the kids and provide many "family favorites" in the recipes in appendix A.

What Is a Lean Meat?

When choosing meat, consider its fat, saturated fat, and cholesterol content per serving, as follows.

Extra lean. Extra lean meat has less than 5 grams of fat, less than 2 grams of saturated fat, and less than 95 milligrams of cholesterol.

Lean. Lean meat has less than 10 grams of fat, less than 4.5 grams of saturated fat, and less than 95 milligrams of cholesterol.

Lean Protein Sources

Lean protein comes in many forms besides chicken and beef. Here's a list of good sources.

Beans

Beef—lean cuts

Chicken—skinless, white meat

Cottage cheese

Eggs (limit yolks to 3 or 4 a week)

Energy bars or shakes—those with less than 25 grams of carbohydrates, fewer than 200 calories, and 2 or more grams of fiber

Fish

Hot dogs—turkey or vegetarian

Legumes

Milk—1% or fat-free

Pork loin

Protein powder

Shellfish (limit shrimp intake if you have high cholesterol)

Turkey—white meat

Veggie burgers and meatballs—those with 5 to 7 grams of protein per ounce

Remember, eating optimum amounts of high-quality protein is a key to success. By increasing the amount of lean protein in your diet, you and your family can control your health and fitness and take charge of weight management.

WHAT'S SO FISHY ABOUT FISH?

Even though fish is a healthy choice for you and your family, some types can be high in mercury. Use this list as a short guide to choosing safe fish fare for your family.

Low in mercury—eat up to 12 ounces a week:

Catfish

Cod

Halibut

Salmon, wild

Shrimp

Tuna, light, canned

Moderately high in mercury—eat no more than 6 ounces a week:

Tuna, albacore (white)

High in mercury—avoid these types:

King mackerel

Shark

Swordfish

Tilefish

PRINCIPLE 4

Add Fiber and Switch to Complex Carbohydrates

America has gone low-carb crazy! Anyone who follows the news has heard the differing opinions about carbohydrates and what we should be eating. My goal is to sort it out for you so that you can design a prudent and healthy meal plan for your family.

Carbohydrates include fruits, dairy products, starches, and starchy vegetables such as potatoes, peas, and corn. Ultimately, carbohydrates break down in your body and become glucose, or sugar. Sugar is also a carbohydrate; therefore, all "sugary" foods are included in this category. Of course, candy, sweets, and sweetened cereals should be limited in your meal plan. Although limiting these sugary foods sounds like a very difficult task, especially for your kids, you will find that your cravings actually decrease as you stop eating them.

I always encourage my clients to choose complex carbohydrates for their meal plans. Complex carbohydrates include foods such as whole grain breads, brown rice, whole wheat pasta, and oatmeal. The fiber content of these foods helps fill you up, and it helps keep your blood sugar levels more stable, thus minimizing sugar cravings. Complex carbohydrates are also good sources of vitamins, minerals, phytonutrients, and antioxidants, and a diet high in them has been linked to the prevention of diabetes, heart disease, and certain cancers. Focusing on the fiber content is one of the easiest ways to differentiate between simple and complex carbohydrates. It's simple: Complex carbohydrates have more fiber, and refined carbs have less.

In addition to promoting foods high in complex carbohydrates, I also recommend limiting refined carbohydrates, which include desserts and sweets as well as refined foods such as white rice, white pasta, and white bread. A diet high in refined carbohydrates has been linked to an increased risk of diabetes, heart disease, and certain cancers. Refined carbohydrates can also contribute to blood sugar fluctuations, which lead to more sugar cravings and overeating.

SENA SAYS:
Don't just be concerned about the *quantity* of carbohydrates; remember to focus on the *quality* of them.

A recent study found that children given high-fiber foods for breakfast felt less hungry and ate less food at lunch. So rather than giving your kids apple juice or even applesauce, have them eat whole apples, which provide not only the juice but also the fiber they'll need to curb their appetite. Now imagine what might happen if *every* meal and snack that you ate included a good fiber source: Everything would fill you up. The more fiber you eat, the fewer calories you'll consume overall!

Another important health benefit of fiber is the way it helps keep your gastrointestinal tract functioning properly. Whether it's soluble fiber (found in oatmeal, potatoes, bananas, soy, and applesauce) or insoluble fiber (from whole grains, nuts, oranges, pears, apples, legumes, and many vegetables), it all helps prevent constipation, hemorrhoids, diverticular disease (painful outpouching of the colon wall), and slow digestion.

HOW MUCH FIBER DO WE NEED?

Unfortunately, the average American consumes only about 14 grams of fiber a day. As you can see from the following chart, it's recommended that we eat a lot more than that.

AGE	RECOMMENDED FIBER INTAKE (GRAMS/DAY)
1–3 years	19
4–8 years	25
Boys, 9–13 years	31
Girls, 9–13 years	26
Teens and adults	25–35

If you find that you're not eating enough fiber, you just need to add some high-fiber foods to your diet. As you can see from the chart below, there are many delicious foods that are considered to be high in fiber.

FOOD	PORTION SIZE	FIBER (GRAMS)
Apple	1 medium	3
Brown rice	⅓ cup	2
Cheerios	¾ cup	3
Kashi Go Lean cereal	¾ cup	10
Kidney beans	½ cup	5
Oatmeal	½ cup	4
Spinach	1 cup	4
Strawberries and other berries	1 cup	3–4
Whole grain breads	1 slice	2–4

FRUITS AND VEGETABLES

Another great way to add more fiber to your diet is to eat more fruits and vegetables. The National Cancer Institute recommends that Americans eat five to nine servings of fruits and vegetables every single day. Along with being high in fiber, fruits and vegetables contain vitamins, minerals, and other phytonutrients that offer an abundance of health benefits. A diet high in fruits and vegetables can prevent cancer, protect you from heart disease and stroke, lower your blood pressure, control your blood sugar, and decrease your risk of cataracts and macular degeneration. In addition, their low caloric value—50 calories per cup of vegetables and 120 per cup of fruit—helps to keep you trim!

LEAN MOM FACT:
The National Cancer Institute has recommended that Americans eat five to nine servings of fruits and vegetables a day.

Unfortunately, many of us fall short of the minimum five-a-day goal. And if *we* fall short of that goal, it's easy to see why many of our kids don't get enough fruit or veggies in their diets. In Week 4, I'll give you some great tips to help you incorporate more fruits and vegetables into your family's daily meal plans.

PRINCIPLE 5

Choose the Right Fats

It amazes me when I see boxes of candy (almost pure sugar) at the movie theater that are labeled as low-fat foods—as if that makes jelly beans or licorice a health food! But the candy companies realized that we've been incorrectly taught that fat is bad and low-fat is good, even if low-fat means eating too much sugar. I'm here to fill you in on a secret: Fat is not the enemy.

In fact, my plan does away with the notion that you must remove fat from your diet. Instead, I'll show you the differences between healthy fats and unhealthy fats. By including certain "good" fats in your meal plans, you will naturally feel full and gain important health benefits.

THE GOOD, THE BAD, AND THE UGLY

The good: unsaturated fats. The healthy fats are known as unsaturated fats, both monounsaturated and polyunsaturated. Monounsaturated fats have been shown to help lower cholesterol and triglyceride levels, lower LDL cholesterol (the bad type), and improve blood sugar levels. Foods that are high in monounsaturated fats include olive oil, canola oil, avocados, and nuts such as almonds.

Polyunsaturated fats are found in foods containing sunflower, safflower, and corn oils. Polyunsaturated fats can also be high in omega-3 fatty acids. These are known as essential fatty acids; your body needs them, yet it cannot produce them, so you must get them from your diet. Omega-3s are very beneficial for lowering cholesterol and triglycerides, decreasing blood pressure, and stabilizing blood sugar levels, and they have even been shown to be helpful for mild depression. Foods high in omega-3s include fatty fish (salmon, sardines, tuna), flaxseeds, flaxseed oil, pumpkin seeds, and walnuts.

LEAN MOM FACT:
Foods high in omega-3 fatty acids include fatty fish (salmon, sardines, tuna), flaxseeds, flaxseed oil, pumpkin seeds, and walnuts.

One thing to remember: Fats are very high in calories. I am not recommending that you drink olive oil or eat pounds of almonds! Watch your portion sizes: A serving of oil is 1 teaspoon, and six to eight almonds will give you all the healthy fats you need.

The bad: saturated fats. Saturated fat is the fat that can contribute to high cholesterol and triglyceride levels. It's found in animal products, including butter, eggs, lard, beef, pork, poultry (particularly in the skin and dark meat), processed meats (such as salami, sausage, and pepperoni), and whole-fat dairy products (such as whole milk and ice cream).

FOOD	PORTION SIZE	SATURATED FAT (GRAMS)
American cheese	1 oz	5.6
Egg	1 large	1.7
Eye of round, roasted	4 oz	2.5
Hamburger, 90% lean	4 oz	8.0
Ice cream	1 cup	14.0
Pork tenderloin	4 oz	2.0
Salami	1 slice	2.0
Spareribs	4 oz	14.0

The ugly: hydrogenated fats (trans fats). Hydrogenated fats, also known as trans fats, have been shown to be even more hazardous to your health than saturated fats because they increase your LDL (bad) cholesterol and decrease your HDL (good) cholesterol. Most fried foods tend to be prepared in hydrogenated or partially hydrogenated oils. These unhealthy fats are also found in processed and prepared foods such as cookies, crackers, chips, snack foods, muffins, pastries, frozen waffles, and frozen dinners. The FDA has mandated that all food labels list the amount of hydrogenated fats in a food by 2006.

SENA SAYS:
Limit the amount of foods you eat that have hydrogenated fats, partially hydrogenated fats, or shortening listed in the ingredients.

Margarines can contain hydrogenated fats, but for a healthier option, look for one that says "No trans fats" on the label. Butter is still a better choice because it doesn't contain the chemicals that are usually found in margarine. Ideally, try mixing butter and olive oil in a small bowl for a spread that has the taste of butter with the health benefits of monounsaturated fat.

The American Heart Association recommends limiting hydrogenated and saturated fats to no more than 7 to 10 percent of your daily calories, depending on your cholesterol levels. If you're following a 1,700-calorie diet, you should eat no more than 13 to 17 grams of saturated and hydrogenated fats each day.

FOOD	PORTION SIZE	TRANS FATS (GRAMS)
Candy	3 oz	6.9
Cheese cracker sandwiches	6	2.8
Fast-food french fries	3 oz	1.0–5.0
Microwave popcorn	3.5-oz bag	8.8
Muffin	3 oz	3.0

PRINCIPLE 6

Calories Still Count

In recent years, calories have not been given the attention they deserve. We've moved away from calorie counting and instead have become obsessed with cutting fat, and now carbs, from our diets. When fat was taken out of foods, sugar was added, and when carbohydrates were taken out of our diets, fat was added. So we've gone from snacking on whole boxes of fat-free cookies to eating huge platters of bacon and steak! In the end, we are still consuming too many calories and not burning off enough of them through activity.

Don't worry; I'm not bringing back strict calorie counting. Instead, I just want you to work toward a good balance of complex carbohydrates, lean protein, and fruits and vegetables while keeping an eye on portion size.

Limiting the number of poor-quality calories we consume is crucial to maintaining a good balance of the nutrients our bodies need. Americans currently spend 90 percent of their food dollar on processed foods—a good reflection of the state of our nutritional health. Nearly one-third of our children's diets contain high-calorie, low-nutrient foods. In general, processed foods (which include most fast foods and junk foods) tend to be high in saturated fats and hydrogenated fats, low in fiber, lacking in fruits and vegetables, and low in nutrients. Stocking your refrigerator and pantry with whole, unprocessed foods will make your goals of a healthy weight and a healthy body much easier to attain.

LEAN MOM FACT:
Americans currently spend 90 percent of their food dollar on processed foods.

PRINCIPLE 7

You Are What You Drink

It may seem as if it will be an uphill battle to get your family to switch from heavily advertised sodas, energy drinks, and sugary juice drinks to healthier beverages such as water and milk. Believe me, though, it's a battle worth fighting.

The high intake of these sugar-sweetened drinks has been a driving force behind the high incidence of obesity among our children. Did you know that one 12-ounce can of soda has *10 teaspoons of sugar*? I'm sure that none of you would knowingly give that much sugar to your kids with their meals or snacks.

Soda drinkers are also more likely to have a lower intake of important nutrients, such as vitamin C, vitamin A, folate, magnesium, and calcium. The decrease in calcium can result in reduced bone mass, which can contribute to broken bones in children and can possibly lead to osteoporosis later in life.

There are two ways to win this battle. One is to make sure everyone understands just how dangerous sugary drinks can be. Let

LEAN MOM FACT:
A study of more than 500 children ages 11 and 12 found that a child's chance of becoming obese increased 60 percent for every sugar-sweetened drink he consumed each day.

your kids and spouse know that these drinks are leading culprits in weight gain and dental problems and how the lack of dairy-based drinks can lead to broken bones.

The other necessary tactic is to provide healthier choices that your family will learn to love.

SOFT DRINKS = LIQUID CANDY = WEIGHT GAIN

If you or anyone else in your family is looking to lose weight, there is no better place to start than by cutting out soft drinks, which are nothing more than liquid candy. I have had many clients lose between 5 and 10 pounds just by reducing the amount of sugar-sweetened beverages they consumed. Here is an example of how these calories can add up in a typical day.

Breakfast	12 ounces of orange juice	150 calories
Lunch	King-size soda	430 calories
Afternoon	12-ounce can of regular soda	150 calories
Dinner	12-ounce fruit drink	150 calories
		Total 880 calories

On the other hand, reducing your intake as shown in the example below can save 520 calories a day—which amounts to a 1-pound weight loss in 1 week!

Breakfast	8 ounces of orange juice	100 calories
Lunch	Small soda	160 calories
Afternoon	Water or unsweetened iced tea with lemon	0 calories
Dinner	8 ounces of low-fat milk	100 calories
		Total 360 calories

GOOD DRINK OPTIONS YOUR FAMILY WILL ENJOY

As you are convincing your family to decrease their sugary drink intake, you can introduce them to these better choices.

Water. Whether it is flat or fizzy, flavored or plain, water is a fundamental component of your family fitness plan and is the *perfect* beverage for everyone. It helps to fill you up and is important for many bodily functions. There are many drinks masquerading as water that still have sugar or artificial sweeteners added. Check to be sure the label lists no calories or artificial sweeteners so you get the real deal. Show your kids that the ever-present water bottles that lots of pro athletes, teenagers, and health-conscious young adults carry with them are healthy and cool! Here are some ideas for making water more appealing to your kids.

❏ Have plenty of flavored seltzer waters available as an alternative to plain water.

❏ Use fresh lemon, lime, or other citrus fruit slices in your water. Or try cucumber slices for a refreshing taste.

❏ Always keep water bottles in the car or in your kids' backpacks to encourage water consumption.

Milk. Low-fat and fat-free milk are healthful beverage alternatives. Next to water, low-fat or fat-free milk and soy milk are the best beverage options for your family. Milk contains calcium, which we often don't get enough of, as well as protein. Soy milk is a great alternative to cow's milk, especially if you are lactose intolerant, have problems with chronic upper respiratory infections (sinus infections or ear infections), have asthma, or are just looking to include more soy in your diet. Chocolate

LEAN MOM FACT:
Only 32 percent of boys ages 12 to 19, 12 percent of girls ages 12 to 19, and 11 to 16 percent of adult women get the daily recommended amount of calcium.

milk is okay for an occasional treat; just try to control the amount of chocolate added to keep the sugar under control.

100 percent fruit juice. 100 percent fruit juice is just that—it is made solely from fruit with no sugar added. Fruit juice has the added benefit of being full of the vitamins that are naturally found in fruit, such as vitamin C and folate. It's very important to remember, however, that a serving is only 4 ounces. The typical juice box is 8 ounces, and many bottles can be up to 20 ounces. I would suggest limiting the total amount of juice for the day to 4 to 8 ounces. If 8 ounces is much less than your family is used to drinking, dilute the juice with water. Start with 25 percent water and 75 percent juice, then slowly increase the percentage of water to 50 percent. Or try mixing juice with seltzer water for a fizzy treat.

Vegetable juice. Vegetable juice is a great low-calorie choice that offers antioxidants, such as vitamins A and C, and other nutrients such as lycopene, which has been linked to a reduced risk of prostate cancer. Eight ounces of vegetable juice has 2 grams of fiber, is very low in sugar, and has only 50 calories.

Unsweetened teas. Unsweetened teas—those that are already bottled—and homemade iced or hot herbal teas can be great calorie-free options. Black and green teas also have proven health benefits, such as decreasing your risk of cancer and lowering cholesterol. Many herbal teas taste sweet enough on their own, so you don't need to add any extra sugar or honey. If they don't, try adding a small amount of 100 percent fruit juice for a delicious blend. Teas come in many family-friendly flavors, such as berry, orange, and cinnamon, so you have plenty of options to try. When buying bottled teas, be sure to check the nutrition labels to make certain they have no calories.

Sports drinks. Sports drinks are very popular among kids, due in large part to great marketing and advertisements. Sports drinks contain only about 50 to 80 calories per 8 ounces, making them lower in calories than juices, fruit drinks, and soda. They don't, however, offer the nutritional benefits of 100 percent fruit juice, vegetable juice, or milk—so drink them only occasionally. Water is still the best fluid choice for any activity that lasts less than 60 minutes, making it ideal for a typical workout. Water also won't replace the calories that you're working to burn off!

BEST AND WORST DRINK CHOICES FOR YOUR FAMILY

DRINK	WHAT'S GOOD	WHAT'S NOT SO GOOD	VERDICT
Water	Helps fill you up with no calories	It's all good	Best choice
Flavored water	Water is good, and everybody likes a little flavor	Watch that it doesn't contain calories or artificial sweeteners	Just as good as plain water, but with a flair
Vitamin water	Lower in calories than other drinks; contains nutrients	Not as good as the real deal	Good in moderation
Sports drinks	Lower in calories and good for hydrating during workouts longer than 60 minutes	Don't contain any vitamins or other nutrients	Good in moderation
100% juice	Contains vitamin C and folate	Contains naturally occurring sugar from fruit	Good in moderation (limit to 4–8 ounces a day)

DRINK	WHAT'S GOOD	WHAT'S NOT SO GOOD	VERDICT
Organic juice	Free of herbicides and pesticides; good for environment	Contains naturally occurring sugar from fruit	Good in moderation (same limit as 100% juice)
Juice drinks such as Hawaiian Punch, Kool-Aid, Tang, Snapple	Not too much is good about these drinks	Very high in added sugar with no nutrients	Try to eliminate, or limit to 1 or 2 times a month
Lemonade	Not too much is good unless homemade with real lemons and a limited amount of added sugar	High in added sugar with no nutrients (unless homemade with real lemons)	Try to limit to 1 or 2 times a month
Diet drinks	No calories	Contain artificial sweeteners	Limit to occasional use
Vegetable juice	Good source of vitamins A and C; low in calories; contains some fiber	High in sodium	Good snack to help fill you up
Unsweetened tea	No calories	No nutrients	Good alternative to water
Sweetened tea	Not too good unless homemade with a limited amount of added sugar	High in added sugar	Try to eliminate, or limit to 1 or 2 times a month
Soda	Not too much is good about soda	High in added sugar and caffeine	Try to eliminate, or limit to 1 or 2 times a month
Milk	Great source of calcium, vitamin D, and protein	Whole milk and 2% milk contain saturated fat	Great drink choice and calcium source
Chocolate milk	Great source of calcium, vitamin D, and protein	High in sugar	Limit to occasional treat
Soy milk	Great source of calcium, vitamin D, and soy protein	Some people have an aversion to the taste of soy milk	Great drink choice and calcium source

OTHER DRINKS

Perhaps some of your favorite drinks aren't described above—and for good reason. Here's the skinny on some other popular drinks that you'll want to avoid.

Diet soda. My tendency is to recommend eating real foods and avoiding artificial sweeteners and fat replacements, such as aspartame and Olestra. Aspartame, a common sweetener in diet soda, has been linked to migraine headaches, among other adverse health reactions. In addition, there is a small amount of preliminary research indicating that your body releases insulin in response to artificial sweeteners. The release of insulin causes your blood sugar levels to drop and therefore makes you hungry. Trying to decrease the amount of sweeteners you use, whether they're natural or chemical, is the best bet. However, allow yourself to enjoy your favorite sweet occasionally, made with real sugar. If you choose to drink diet soda or use artificial sweeteners, do so in moderation (once or twice a week).

> ## SODA IN SCHOOLS
>
> As of this writing, there are many school districts around the country that have realized they have been inadvertently contributing to the obesity problem through the foods they offer in their cafeterias and vending machines. School districts in Chicago, San Francisco, and New York City have made healthy changes to their cafeteria menus and are eliminating soda and other high-fat, high-sugar vending-machine foods and replacing them with healthier alternatives. We applaud their efforts!
>
> If you are interested in making changes in your local school system, check out th Web site www.actionforhealthykids.org.

Coffee drinks. With the rise of the chain coffee houses has come the popularity of creamy coffee drinks that are chock full of sugar and calories. A 16-ounce café mocha averages 300 to 350 calories, while a 16-ounce frozen coffee drink can have anywhere from 300 to more than 500 calories, depending on what "extras" you have added. Whipped cream alone can add more than 100 calories! Bakery treats such as banana bread, muffins, and scones have, on average, between 350 and 450 calories, while a caramel sticky roll or slice of coffee cake can have upwards of 700 calories. Yikes! You could easily get more than half of your daily calorie allowance from your coffee break.

Fortunately, you don't have to forgo your treat. There are many lower-calorie choices, such as a small café latte or cappuccino made with fat-free milk (about 120 calories). You could also try a 12-ounce Chai tea with fat-free milk for about 170 calories. Choose from a selection of herbal teas or, of course, plain old zero-calorie black java. And instead of the muffins or cake, try a crunchy biscotti for around 120 calories.

Alcohol. Alcohol is another underestimated calorie source. A 12-ounce beer, a 7-ounce glass of wine, or a 2.5-ounce martini each adds around 150 empty calories. And that can double if you're drinking a tall glass of a creamy mixer such as piña colada. Also, alcohol tends to lower your inhibitions, so

LEAN MOM FACT:
You can easily reach one-third to one-half of your daily calorie quota with a stop at the coffee shop for a medium café mocha and a blueberry muffin.

you are more likely to take a few extra bites of dessert. In addition to contributing to extra weight, alcohol has been shown to have differing effects on your health. Moderate amounts of red wine (one drink a day for women and two drinks a day for men) have been shown to lower the risk of coronary heart disease. However, research has also shown that alcohol in higher amounts can be a contributor to cancers of the breast, esophagus, stomach, and colon. Use judgment and moderation when fitting alcohol into your meal plan.

ON TO THE 6-WEEK PLAN

You now have the educational foundation to move into Week 1 and the beginning of the action part of my plan. As we go through each week, you will notice that the seven principles we just reviewed are emphasized throughout. Understanding and incorporating these guidelines into your daily family meals and snacks are crucial to a healthy weight and a healthy heart—and the keys to feeling energized, strong, and fit!

PART 2

The Lean Mom, Fit Family 6-Week Plan

Here is where fun meets fitness. We're about to put my Seven Principles of Family Fitness into action with you and your family. Together, we'll take a 6-week journey that will reshape your waistline—and your family's everyday health habits.

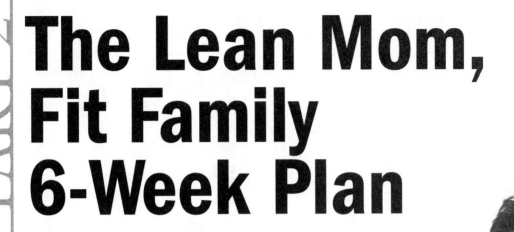

Getting Started, Step by Step

Having seen other families transformed by my plan, I'm confident that we'll get the job done in 6 weeks. I know that you have a few (hundred!) things going on in your life other than this plan, but I ask you, is there anything more important than your family's health?

JUST FOR YOU, MOM

Before we start the family program, I want to share a few thoughts just for you, Mom. I'm going to continue this one-on-one dialogue throughout the book, and each week will have a section that addresses you and your feelings.

I understand that before you can take a leading role in your family's fitness, you have to feel good about the way you look and feel. You also have to figure out how to juggle your busy life to find time to focus on this plan.

I promise, as you start taking the steps outlined in this book, you will begin moving in the direction of your target weight. It may happen more gradually than you desire, or it may happen faster than you anticipated. Either way, it's great, because once you get started, you're going to keep moving down the path toward your goals. Just a little success will buoy your spirits and propel you forward. Ultimately, you'll be able to help the rest of your family members achieve their objectives as well.

I also am very aware that I am asking you for the thing that is the most scarce in your life—your time. But I know that you'll find that getting fit takes very little time every day. This plan is all about making small changes, a few at a time. Those small changes will add up to big results at the end of 6 weeks. So circle the date on your calendar 6 weeks from now and believe with all your heart that you will look and feel wonderful when that date comes.

ORGANIZE A FAMILY KICKOFF MEETING

Before you get started, I'd like to go over a few things to set you and your family up for success. You will want to schedule a Kickoff Meeting. Think of this as your preseason training camp. It's the Kickoff Meeting that gets everyone in your family ready for their 6-week success story. Once each member of your family has signed off on their participation in the program and has gone through the steps outlined below, you'll be ready to start the plan.

The purpose of your Kickoff Meeting is to establish health baselines for each family member, define commitments, target goals, outline strategies, and agree on time frames for actions and results. In other words, you want to have all family members be aware of their current health and fitness status (acceptance), decide what they want to improve upon (goal setting), and determine how to accomplish those goals (strategy).

The Kickoff Meeting will also set the stage for future Fit Family Meetings throughout the program. At the start of every week, you'll want to hold a Fit Family Meeting to discuss progress and potential setbacks and to talk about the program. Each week, as you move through the program, I'll give you an agenda for your meeting. It's a time for everyone to prepare themselves for success.

You want your family members to grasp the fact that what they do in their lives now will be reflected in their health status in years to come. You must communicate how much you care: You love them and want them to enjoy a life with more good health, happiness, energy, and achievement. I want you to also stress the importance of the family support system and how all family members will do this together, encourage one another, and answer to the family as a whole. For a family fitness plan to work best, the *entire* family must be present and be involved.

Here are the things that you will cover in your Kickoff Meeting. Just schedule 90 minutes together (maybe along with a healthy Sunday brunch) and go through the following steps, in order, one at a time. As a reminder, as stated in the introduction to this book, you should have all received medical clearance before you have your Kickoff Meeting.

KICKOFF MEETING AGENDA

1. Adopt the right attitude and commit to success.
2. Develop your family fitness profile.
3. Set goals.
4. Determine strategies to meet your goals.
5. Commit to keeping food diaries.
6. Commit to using exercise/activity journals.
7. Schedule your Week 1 Fit Family Meeting.

STEP 1: ADOPT THE RIGHT ATTITUDE AND COMMIT TO SUCCESS

The longer I live, the more I realize the impact of attitude on life. Attitude to me is more important than education, genius, experience, or the facts! —*Charles Swindoll*

These inspiring words epitomize the definition of what a positive attitude is all about. I suggest that you begin your Kickoff Meeting by reading this quote out loud. It will help get everyone in a positive and empowered frame of mind so they have the right attitude about getting healthy and fit! People who don't concern themselves with their mental outlook, and who think they have the answers or the know-how, often underestimate attitude. This is a huge mistake. If you don't have a positive attitude about what you're striving for and why you are doing it, you will never get there—plain and simple. Let me share with you the best example of a positive attitude that I have seen in recent times. I encourage you to share this story with your family as your Kickoff Meeting gets under way. Start by asking your kids if they know the story of Lance Armstrong. Maybe they can tell this story to you!

Lance Armstrong is a world-class cyclist who has now won six straight Tour de France races, a feat never before accomplished. Amazing, wouldn't you say? Yes, but to me, it pales in comparison to the fact that before winning these six races, he was diagnosed with cancer, went through surgery, underwent radiation treatment, made a full recovery, and was back on his bike in less than a year. Wow! Can you imagine the kind of attitude a person must possess when he is told that he has cancer, stands up to it, defeats it, and then achieves an epic goal? A 100 percent *positive* attitude is the only way to describe it! Ever since I learned of Lance's comeback, I have attempted to emulate his outlook and attitude when reaching toward my own goals, and I ask you to do the same.

You don't have to go for world records. You just need to commit to having a positive and healthy impact on your world. Be grateful that you have the ability and opportunity to change an important part of your life and your family members' lives. Live with passion, be positive, and be successful!

Ready to take your new attitude for a test drive? Start by converting your positive attitude into something very tangible—*commitment*. As I have always told people who come to me for guidance regarding their health and fitness, "You must make a real, strong, and honest commitment to yourself that you will do whatever it takes to achieve your goals." The absence of this commitment will set you up for failure 100 percent of the time. I know, because I have failed myself. Are there some days when you oversleep or don't work out as long as you wanted? Times when you eat a bowl of ice cream, even though you had promised yourself that you wouldn't? As long as you have made a strong commitment, you can work through those little failures and reach your goals.

Make sure that your family understands that commitment is the glue that keeps it together when things get tough or when you want to quit. Let commitment be your guide down the path of your family's journey to success. Once everyone in your family commits, there's no question that they will stick to it. And if they stick to it, they will succeed.

STEP 2: DEVELOP YOUR FAMILY FITNESS PROFILE

Once you have the right attitude, and you have made your commitment, it's time to put your plan in motion. The first thing you need to do, for yourself and for your family, is to establish your starting point.

The following is a list of questions that I have developed for you to use to get an accurate indication of the fitness and health habits of yourself and each member of your family. It also lets you know what the road ahead will look like as you start my plan to bring you optimum health. In no way are these questions designed to take the place of your doctor's advice or medical clearance. As stated previously, you should always get your doctor's approval before beginning this or any other health and fitness program.

Make photocopies of the Fit Family Quiz on page 36, pass them out at the meeting, and have everyone fill out their own. Walk younger kids through the quiz one question at a time to make sure they understand everything.

Each member of your family should answer honestly and accurately. You should keep a record of each family member's scores in order to provide specific focus and direction. For example, if you see that your teenage daughter is drinking lots of sugary beverages but very little water, that will be an initial point of focus. Or if you notice that your husband is eating very little fiber and getting very little cardiovascular exercise, you may want to focus on initiating an early-morning routine of a brisk walk followed by a bowl of whole grain cereal with fresh fruit. Once each family member's baseline is established, you can support and guide each other toward optimum health. The more family members who have a healthy lifestyle, the better off you all will be—because those healthy individuals can play a key role of support and lead by example.

FIT FAMILY QUIZ

Ask each family member this series of questions and insert their total score in the chart on page 38.

1. How often do you eat at fast-food restaurants?

   Once a week = 1   Twice a week = 3

   Three or more times a week = 5

2. Do you take daily vitamins?

   Yes = 1   Sometimes = 2   No = 3

3. Do you smoke?

   No = 1   Sometimes = 3   Yes = 5

4. How many meals do you skip each day?

   0 = 1   1 = 2   2 or more = 4

5. How many glasses of water do you drink daily?

   6 to 8 = 1   3 to 5 = 3   0 to 2 = 5

6. How many servings of fiber do you eat daily?

   4 or 5 = 1   2 or 3 = 3   0 to 1 = 5

7. How many sugar-sweetened beverages do you drink daily?

   0 or 1 = 1   2 = 3   3 or more = 5

8. How many sugary treats do you eat per day?

   0 or 1 = 1   2 or 3 = 3   3 or more = 5

9. Do you drink alcohol? How much?

   0 or 1 drink per day = 1   2 or 3 drinks per day = 4

   3+ drinks per day = 5

10. How many servings of fruits and vegetables do you eat each day?

    4 or 5 = 1   2 or 3 = 2   0 or 1 = 4

11. Do you eat in response to stress or other emotions?

    No = 1   Sometimes = 3   Yes = 5

12. Do you eat fried foods more than two times per week?

    No = 1   Sometimes = 3   Yes = 5

13. How often do you eat fresh fish?

    3 to 5 times/week = 1   1 or 2 times/week = 3   0 times/week = 5

14. How close are you to your ideal body weight?

    Within 5 pounds = 1   6 to 10 pounds over = 3
    11 or more pounds over = 5

15. Do you eat healthy snacks (fruit and veggies)?

    Yes = 1   Sometimes = 2   No = 3

16. Do you have low energy levels and/or severe mood swings throughout the day?

    No = 1   Sometimes = 3   Yes = 5

17. How often do you engage in cardiovascular activities?

    5 days/week = 1   2 to 4 days/week = 3   0 or 1 day/week = 5

18. How often do you strength train?

    4 or more times/week = 1   2 or 3 times/week = 3   0 or 1 time/week = 5

19. How often do you take part in fun, healthy family activities and outings?

    At least 2 times/month = 1   1 time/month = 2
    Every 2 to 3 months = 3   Every 5 to 8 months = 5

20. How many hours do you sleep each night?

    8 to 10 = 1   6 to 7 = 3   5 or less = 5

Now add up the points to determine each family member's Fit Family Quiz score.

SCORING

20 to 30: Excellent! You're doing great—be a role model for other family members.

31 to 49: Good. You're doing well—stay consistent and look for ways to go to the next level.

50 to 68: Fair. You have plenty of room for improvement—evaluate and make adjustments.

69 to 94: Poor. Your health habits create significant health concerns. You need to focus seriously on health and fitness in your life. Consult a physician or other health professional.

Fill in each family member's score below, in the "Starting Score" column, to establish a baseline for their 6-week Lean Mom, Fit Family Program.

NAME	STARTING SCORE	WEEK 4 SCORE	WEEK 6 SCORE
1.			
2.			
3.			
4.			
5.			
6.			

Honest Assessment

Once each family member has answered all 20 questions and everyone has tallied up their scores, your family fitness program will begin to take shape. Remember, accuracy and honesty are the first steps in taking matters into your own hands. Accepting that you do have certain unhealthy habits in your daily routines will make the transition much easier and the program more effective.

Before you go any further, stop and review everyone's evaluation with the entire family. (You'll want everyone to keep the forms as a reference throughout the program.) Go over each question to see how everyone is doing, one issue at a time. What have you discovered? Does your whole family drink too much soda? Eat too few fruits and vegetables? As a parent and caretaker of the family, you'll want to help everyone understand where they stand, what the information means, and why the situation needs to improve. If necessary, a health professional such as your family doctor can assist you with interpretations of the findings. This is a crucial first step!

STEP 3: SET GOALS

After you have discussed where each person is, and you have a sense of which areas need the most work, it is time to go around the room and ask each family member to write down their goals and what strategies they'll use to reach those goals. Fitness goals, in large part, should be created to improve individual evaluation scores over the duration of the 6-week program.

Goal setting is one of the most significant and necessary acts that we perform each day to organize our lives as we move forward toward our dreams and passions. Goal setting helps us stay focused on the prize as we strive to reach what we want in our lives. Regardless of who you are and whether you're young, old, thin, heavy, poor, or rich, at the end of the day, you will be no farther along the road of progress if your day didn't start with writing down your goals in order of priority.

There are important *short-term* goals and *long-term* goals that must be handled properly if your ultimate dreams are to be realized. Don't confuse the two. Long-term goals are big goals, such as losing 20 pounds, making the basketball team, or being healthier. Short-term goals are smaller, such as going for a walk 3 days a week, learning to strength train, or drinking more water. As you set smaller goals and achieve them, before you know it, all those small goals will add up to one big success. It works like a charm.

Examples of Fitness Goals for Adults

❏ Lose weight

❏ Build lean muscle

❏ Decrease body fat percentage

❏ Become more active

❏ Improve function and balance

❏ Get stronger

❏ Build endurance

❏ Learn how to cook healthfully

❏ Lower bad cholesterol

❏ Lower blood pressure

❏ Lower risk of heart disease and diabetes

❏ Feel younger

❏ Take inches off your waistline

❏ Tone up your muscles

❏ Alleviate back pain

Examples of Fitness Goals for Children

- ❏ Eat healthier snacks
- ❏ Learn a new sport or activity (jump rope, soccer, gymnastics, swimming)
- ❏ Watch less TV
- ❏ Reduce time with video games
- ❏ Increase time devoted to fitness activities
- ❏ Eliminate trips to fast-food restaurants
- ❏ Avoid candy vending machines
- ❏ Learn more about healthy food versus unhealthy food
- ❏ Become part of an organized sports team
- ❏ Drink more water and less soda

Each family member should now list his or her top five goals using a photocopy of the following blank log. Here's an example.

Name: _____ Mary _____

Long-Term Goal: Lose 20 to 40 pounds

Short-Term Goal #1: Lose 1 to 2 pounds per week

Short-Term Goal #2: Improve cardiovascular health

Short-Term Goal #3: Play sports without getting tired so fast

Short-Term Goal #4: Feel healthier; lower cholesterol

Now, here's the form to copy.

FITNESS GOAL LOG

Name: _____

Long-Term Goal: _____

Short-Term Goal #1: _____

Short-Term Goal #2: _____

Short-Term Goal #3: _____

Short-Term Goal #4: _____

STEP 4: DETERMINE STRATEGIES TO MEET YOUR GOALS

With everyone's goal lists firmly in hand, it's time to go around the room and have each family member write down their strategies.

Even with a positive attitude, strong commitment, and short- and long-term goals clearly stated and documented, you still need direction and a road map of how you will reach your ultimate goals. That's where strategizing comes in. Your strategies need to get right down to what days you will exercise, planning your food menu for the week, and even how much sleep you'll need to be healthy and strong for the challenges ahead.

You must have your goals and strategies very clearly defined. *Goals* are what each family member wants to achieve, and *strategies* are how you will achieve them.

For each set of goals that was created in Step 3, now create a method that you will use to reach your goals, the structure of your plan, and exactly what you will need to do in order to be successful. Let's select "lose 20 to 40 pounds" and "reduce the risk of heart disease" as our goals for this example. Strategies for achieving these goals would be the following.

❏ Perform cardiovascular activity 3 to 5 days per week for 20 to 40 minutes per day.

❏ Perform strength-training activity 2 or 3 days per week (total-body workout; approximately 20 to 30 minutes).

❏ Schedule the time of day when the activities will take place and what days of the week you will exercise.

❏ Coordinate time schedules with babysitters and family members so that you can perform your fitness activities.

❏ Determine your meal plan and specific nutritional requirements to lose 20 to 40 pounds.

❏ Decide on and adhere to meal and snack times as well as what foods you will actually eat.

If steps like getting more rest or taking care of an injury through rehabilitation are needed for you to reach your goals, they should be part of your strategy as well. In short, any action or preparation that you or a family member needs to take in order to accomplish a goal is always a part of the strategy. Once established, the goals and strategies are guided and propelled by your commitment—the commitment that each family member has made to himself or herself and to the entire family.

It's important to remember that even the best of plans can sometimes fail. With a strong focus and commitment, you and your family will be able to guide your goals and strategies around the potholes in the road to wellness. You will be able to fight through the times when you do not want to exercise and when you feel like indulging in unhealthy food. Remember, commitment is the cornerstone of every strong marriage, personal relationship, and career, as well as every successful outcome that was worth the effort of forging ahead. Your family's health is definitely worth the effort—so hang in there!

STEP 5: COMMIT TO KEEPING FOOD DIARIES

A food diary is an amazing tool that I assure you will help you reach your weight and fitness goals. I've included a template on the opposite page; photocopy a supply for each of your family members. Everyone should keep a food diary every day for the entire 6-week plan, so be sure to run off plenty of copies. Of course, if you forget to take your form with you, you can use a notebook, a PalmPilot, or even the side of a lunch bag.

When I work with new clients who want to lose weight, the very first question I ask is what they ate in the 3 days before our session. Amazingly, they can usually remember only bits and pieces. Some don't want to remember, or admit, all of the junk that they consumed! Others are so busy that it's a blur.

 SENA SAYS:
Write it down. That is the *only* way you will become aware of what you're eating and really know what needs to change. It's a foolproof tool.

Most of us just don't pay enough attention to what we eat.

The best way to recall what you have eaten—and how much—is to write it down. Keeping a daily log of food and beverages consumed is the *single best way* to approach weight management. Your food diary will help you recognize if you are a healthy eater or not and will tell you just how much food you really are consuming on a daily basis. Once you see it on paper, you can analyze the healthfulness of your diet. Food diaries are critical to the success of your family fitness program.

You can make a lot of progress by filling out your food diaries each day and then reviewing them at the Fit Family Meetings. Together, your family can discuss each other's food diaries by comparing them to the healthy choices outlined in this book. Posting these charts in a central location, such as the kitchen, is a great idea. This "public record" will become a great family conversation piece and a motivator for coaching each other toward success. Remember to support and encourage each other, and don't criticize.

The most significant result of keeping a food diary is self-evaluation and awareness. You may be surprised when you realize how many candy bars and cookies you really ate over the past 7 days. Simply keep a log of what you eat and drink each day, when you eat it, and your feelings at the time. Do your best to recall *everything*, even if it's just a handful or a few pieces of something. It all adds up.

FOOD DIARY NAME _____ DATE _____

MEAL	TYPE AND AMOUNT OF FOOD EATEN	FEELINGS; ENERGY LEVEL (Are you eating in response to hunger? Boredom? Stress?)
Breakfast		
Snack		
Lunch		
Snack		
Dinner		

STEP 6: COMMIT TO USING EXERCISE/ACTIVITY JOURNALS

Now it's time to pass out the exercise/activity journals. Prior to the meeting, make photocopies of the forms on the opposite page. Unlike the food diaries, you'll need only one journal each week for each family member. You don't need to fill in anything yet. Just explain their purpose and make sure everyone understands how to use them and agrees to use them once Week 1 begins.

These journals work like the food diaries. Just write the date and the length of time you were active in the appropriate spaces. You'll see that the journal includes a Fit Family Activity. Each week, I'll give you suggestions for a healthy activity for the whole family. After your family has picked an activity, write it in the appropriate space. As with the food diaries, you'll discuss the week's activity at the Fit Family Meeting.

Writing down your weekly physical activities is a simple and smart method to help you reach your goals. Using an exercise/activity journal is a proven way to stay focused and committed to your goals. By creating a tracking method, you will be able to begin to see your progress from week to week, help create new habits, and discover where adjustments might need to be made. Your exercise/activity journals should be centrally located in the house (maybe in the exercise room or kitchen) for accountability and support. This public showing is fun and gets everyone in the family involved with friendly ribbing and encouragement. You can even foster some friendly family competition with comments such as "C'mon slacker— get the lead out!"

EXERCISE/ACTIVITY JOURNAL

Name: _____

Week of: _____

Fit Family Activity: _____

DAY/DATE	CARDIOVASCULAR EXERCISE (duration)	STRENGTH TRAINING (duration)

Monday

Tuesday

Wednesday

Thursday

Friday

Saturday

Sunday

STEP 7: SCHEDULE YOUR WEEK 1 FIT FAMILY MEETING

The final step of your Kickoff Meeting is easy but important. Take the time now to schedule your Week 1 Fit Family meeting. This is the "official" starting point of your 6-week program. Make sure you find a time that's convenient for everyone—we need the entire family in attendance! Saturday or Sunday is a great time to get everyone together and get focused on the healthy week ahead. See you at your Week 1 meeting!

Wake Up Your Metabolism with Breakfast

Welcome! I hope everyone in your family is excited to be starting on the path to a healthy new lifestyle together. This is an important week.

JUST FOR YOU, MOM

Before we get into the details of Week 1, I'd like to speak to you, Mom. It is important to me that you reach your goals and feel great about yourself as soon as possible. I want you to learn and absorb all that I have perfected over the years to help you achieve your fitness goals.

Sometimes, when we have a bit of a mountain to climb, it can seem insurmountable. But I promise, once you get started, once you accomplish just a little bit of activity, you will immediately feel better, and you will be on your way to success. As soon as you get into your activity for about 5 minutes, you'll feel empowered and motivated to continue. Let's do this together.

You will lose weight this week, Mom, if you:

❑ Cut out all white-flour products, such as bread, pasta, and rice (reduces water retention).

❑ Drink one full 10- to 12-ounce glass of water before each meal (prevents overeating).

❑ Eat some protein at every meal (repairs muscle and helps burn calories).

❑ Do 20 minutes of cardio in the A.M. and 10 to 20 minutes in the P.M. (increases metabolic rate to burn calories at rest). See this week's Fitness Focus on page 71 for ideas for cardio that will fit into your busy schedule.

In your Kickoff Meeting, you established your baselines with your fitness profiles, set your goals and strategies, and committed to journaling your food and exercise. Now that you are prepared to begin your 6-week fitness program, go round up the family, and let's get started with your Week 1 Fit Family Meeting.

WEEK 1 FIT FAMILY MEETING AGENDA

❑ Review your fitness profiles, goals, and strategies.

❑ Put your food diaries and exercise/activity journals into action.

❑ Introduce your family to the Big Purge—cupboard cleaning and new grocery list.

❑ Discuss your meal planning and your Week 1 Food Focus: healthy breakfasts.

❑ Discuss and plan your Week 1 Fitness Focus: cardio exercises.

❑ Plan your Fit Family Activity: Get your kicks.

❑ Schedule your Week 2 Fit Family Meeting.

WEEK 1 FIT FAMILY MEETING

When you sit down with your family, you should have:

❑ The completed fitness profiles for each family member

❑ The completed goal and strategy sheets for each family member

❑ The yet-to-be completed food diaries and exercise/activity journals for each family member

❑ A calendar to plan your fitness activities for the week

When your family is together, begin by thanking everyone for participating and remind them how important this 6-week program is and what fun it is going to be.

Start by distributing the family fitness profiles and goals/strategies sheets that you prepared in your Kickoff Meeting. Discuss what family members think they'll need to meet those goals. For instance, has time been set aside for activity? Have the necessary equipment and materials been obtained? In short: Does everyone have everything they need to be successful? If not, now is the time to take care of it, helping each other as needed. If any obstacles are presented, decide as a family how you can make the kinds of changes required in your lifestyles to overcome them. What can each person do to help the others succeed?

Now hand out the food diaries and review carefully with each family member what they are to do. Remind them that it will be fun to see their eating patterns on paper and that this simple step will turbocharge their fitness results. Seeing everything written down in black and white, even if the choices are not healthy, is an effective way for you and your family to start making better choices in the following weeks. You'll be able to decide which food or meal choices can stay for the upcoming weeks and which ones need to go. Remember, small steps are good. You don't want to change too much at once; make sure that family members feel that they can do this without feeling deprived, so they will be motivated to continue.

Make sure that everyone understands that keeping the diaries should be an everyday event and that they will be reviewed at your next weekly meeting. Everyone can get started by filling in what they have eaten so far today.

After you discuss your food diaries, distribute the exercise/activity journals. Remind everyone how to fill them out. Determine where the journals will be displayed. Explain that you'll be keeping the journals to learn from your lapses and that they're not meant to be used to "grade" family members. Instead, you'll learn what tripped you up if you meant to exercise but didn't. Working overtime, staying late at school unexpectedly, and being tired after a long day are all things that can interfere with meeting our fitness goals. We may not be able to control all of these situations, but we can control how we react. Perhaps you planned to swim for 45 minutes at a neighborhood pool after work, but because you were late leaving work, there wasn't time to do what you planned before the pool closed. Instead of completely skipping your exercise for the day, try to have a "Plan B" ready, so you are still able to do something. Could you swim for 20 minutes before the pool closes? After all, some exercise is better than none. If you are not able to do that, be flexible—instead of swimming, how about a brisk walk around the neighborhood? Or maybe you can work out with an aerobics tape at home or play basketball after dinner.

Now you are ready for the specifics of your Week 1 plan. Mom, lead the group in a discussion of the key Week 1 Food and Fitness Focus points:

❑ Cupboard cleaning

❑ New menu plans and healthy breakfasts

❑ Cardiovascular exercise

❑ Your Fit Family Activity

In detail, go through each key point on the agenda, using the information in the rest of this chapter as your guide. Make sure that you get each family member's commitment to the food and fitness activities, and discuss how each person will schedule the activities into their life.

GET YOUR FAMILY INVOLVED IN THE BIG PURGE

This is one of my favorite parts of the plan because it is action based and so effective. I call it the Big Purge, and it means that it's time to get out the old and bring in the new. Let your family know that during this week and in the following weeks, you are going to go through your cabinets, pantry, refrigerator, and freezer and remove the foods that no longer fit into your family's lifestyle. I know that this is easier said than done, but the positive and inspiring feelings you will get from taking action will definitely supersede any sorrow from saying goodbye to your former saturated-fat friends.

I understand that there are some lifetime favorites in there. But while parting with cookies, cupcakes, and potato chips can cause a bit of short-lived sorrow, the sense of elation from taking control of your weight and your health is well worth it. Candidates for the Big Purge are foods that are high in saturated fats, refined sugars, preservatives, and empty calories. These are the foods that have been in your life in the past and have most likely been holding you back from optimum health and fitness.

At first, you may find some resistance to tossing these treats and objects of cravings, but remember, your family is on a mission of health and fitness. After several weeks, no one will miss the old junk food—and they will be encouraged by how much better they are beginning to look and feel. If you do not feel comfortable discarding food items, give them to a shelter or homeless organization.

The Big Purge is an important part of your transformation into a family that enjoys better health and fitness. However, so I don't confuse anyone, let me state my philosophy on this: Going "cold turkey" with anything rarely works. Some people have the personality to do it, but it doesn't work with most of us—especially me! More important, I don't believe in going about any change that way.

So although cupboard cleaning is essential, I recommend gradually weaning yourself from certain foods that are contributing to weight problems and less-than-optimum health. What we really want to create are new, healthy habits now that you're educated about nutrition. A gradual cutback will be much more effective than an all-or-nothing attitude.

I suggest that you go through the list on page 52 and choose two or three items per week to remove from your home—and your lives. During your Week 1 meeting, ask family members for their ideas on what items should be the first to go.

PLAN YOUR NEW GROCERY LIST

With all that extra room in your cabinets and pantry and with the light shining brightly from the back of the refrigerator, you are now ready to create and use your new grocery list. Your list will center on the new way you plan meals for you and your family. Preparing a menu of meals and snacks for the week is the safest and most effective way to guard against buying the wrong types of foods. By shopping for and selecting only what is needed for your predetermined menu, you will be able to limit or even eliminate bad food choices, thus helping you stay on track for reaching your goals. This is an excellent strategy to get your plan started effectively.

Your new shopping list will contain the food groups and examples of healthy foods that are on the "In" list. Remember, if you buy the wrong foods when you're shopping and place

(continued on page 54)

CUPBOARD CLEANING: OUT WITH THE OLD, IN WITH THE NEW

OUT

High-fat meats

Bologna, salami, pastrami

Duck

Fried meats

Ground beef with more than 15% fat

High-fat cuts of pork and beef, such as chuck

Organ meats, such as liver and kidneys

Pepperoni, sausage, bacon

Poultry: dark meat or meat with skin

"Prime" grade beef

Ribs

High-fat frozen entrées

High-fat soups

Cream-based soups

New England clam chowder

High-fat dairy products

High-fat cheese in large amounts

Whole milk

Refined carbohydrates

Egg noodles

White bread, bagels, rolls, pita bread

White pasta

White rice

Breakfast foods

French toast made with white bread

Granola

High-sugar cereals

Pancakes and waffles

Sugar-sweetened cereals

Processed snack foods

Popcorn with butter or other flavorings

Cheese puffs

Chips (tortilla, potato, etc.)

Snack crackers

Sweets

Cakes

Ice cream

Candy

Cookies

Pastries: doughnuts, croissants

Pies

Vegetables

Fried vegetables

Large amounts of canned vegetables (they often contain high levels of sodium and have fewer nutrients than fresh veggies)

Fats and hydrogenated oils

High-fat dips

Regular margarine

Regular mayonnaise, cream cheese, salad dressings

Shortening, lard

Sugar-sweetened drinks

Soda, fruit drinks

IN

Lean meats*

Baked, broiled, roasted, and grilled meats

Beans: baked beans, kidney beans, chickpeas, split peas, lentils

Fish and shellfish: canned and fresh (limit shellfish if cholesterol is high)

Ground beef or turkey: more than 85% lean

Lean beef and pork: round or loin

Lean lunch meats: turkey, chicken, roast beef, ham

Vegetarian meat options: veggie burgers, hot dogs, meatballs

*See page 11 for info on the fat content of meats

Frozen foods

Frozen lean meats, stir-fry with meat and vegetables

Low-fat frozen entrées (look for 5 grams of fat for every 200 calories)

Soups

Bean soups, such as black bean, lentil, split pea, minestrone, and chili

Low-fat soups, such as chicken vegetable and beef barley

Low-fat dairy products

Cheese (in moderation)

Cottage cheese

Fat-free or 1% milk

Reduced-fat mozzarella sticks

Soy or rice milk

Yogurt (low-sugar)

Snack foods with protein

Energy bars, fruit smoothies, edamame

Hard-cooked eggs (limit to 3 egg yolks/week if cholesterol is high)

Whole grains

Whole wheat bread, bagels, pita bread, rolls; brown rice; whole wheat pasta and grains such as barley and couscous

Breakfast foods

Cream of Wheat

French toast made with whole wheat bread

High-fiber cereals and whole grain cereals

Oatmeal

Pancakes and waffles with 3 or more grams of fiber per serving

Snack foods

Applesauce (no sugar added)

Baked chips

Canned fruit in its own juice

Dried fruit, such as raisins and apricots

Fresh fruits, such as grapes, oranges, berries

Frozen blueberries or grapes

Light microwave popcorn or air-popped popcorn

Nuts, such as almonds, walnuts, pecans

Pretzels

Lower-sugar/lower-fat sweets (with protein)

Chocolate milk made with fat-free milk

Energy bars

Frozen fruit bars

Fruit smoothies

Hot chocolate made with fat-free milk

Portioned frozen yogurt

Portioned low-fat pudding

Vegetables

Frozen vegetables

Raw or steamed veggies

Vegetables as snacks

Baby carrots, pepper slices, cucumber slices, broccoli and cauliflower florets

Fats

Butter (in moderation or mixed with olive oil)

Hummus

Low-fat dip (mix with cottage cheese)

Low-fat mayonnaise, cream cheese, salad dressings (*not* fat-free)

Margarine with no trans fats

Vegetable oils (preferably olive oil)

Beverages

Bottled water

Diet soda in moderation

Iced and hot herbal, black, or green teas

100% juice

Seltzer water, flavored and unflavored

them in your cupboards and refrigerator, there's a pretty good chance you will eat them—and that will keep you from attaining ultimate health. After you have reviewed the meal plans for Week 1 on the following pages, put together your new, healthier shopping list. This new list will help transform your lives!

WEEK 1 FOOD FOCUS: HEALTHY BREAKFASTS

Each week, I will focus on a different meal or snack to give your family ideas on how to add new, healthy, and delicious foods into your meal plans. This week, we'll focus on breakfast. Breakfast really is the most important meal of the day. We know that people who skip breakfast end up consuming more calories than they should the rest of the day. When your body goes without food from a 6:00 P.M. dinner until a noontime lunch the following day, it really puts the brakes on your metabolism. This mechanism dates back to caveman days, when we didn't always know when our next meal was coming. Our bodies learned to store more fat if they perceived a threat of a calorie deficit. Unfortunately, our evolution hasn't quite caught up to the 21st century, so we need to be very careful about food "deprivation" for long periods of time. The healthiest approach is eating small meals and snacks throughout the day, including, of course, breakfast.

Now, I know how absolutely crazy your mornings are. You are trying to get everyone showered, dressed, and hair done, possibly with only one bathroom—and if you have teenagers in the house, forget about it! But making time for breakfast, even if it's something your family can take with them, sets everyone up for a great day—nutritionally, emotionally, educationally, and physically.

Here are some healthy breakfast suggestions.

❏ High-fiber, high-protein cereal with low-fat milk

❏ Protein shake with frozen fruit, milk or plain yogurt, and protein powder

❏ Oatmeal with low-fat milk and protein powder

❏ Egg-white omelet with veggies—tomatoes, mushrooms, peppers, spinach, onions

❏ Breakfast Sandwich (page 237): egg white, low-fat cheese, and vegetarian or low-fat sausage on a whole wheat English muffin

❑ Plain or vanilla yogurt with fresh berries and low-fat granola

❑ Low-fat cheese melted on whole wheat toast

❑ Whole Wheat Pancakes (page 239) or waffles with vegetarian or low-fat sausage (whole grain frozen waffles can be a great quick breakfast)

MEAL PLANS

For each week of the Lean Mom, Fit Family plan, you'll find a menu plan that takes the guesswork out of nutrition planning for your family. The menus have been calculated to provide the proper balance of protein, fat, and carbs and are centered on the Seven Principles of Family Fitness that were described in part 1. Because nonstarchy vegetables are so low in calories, I encourage you to fill up on them. If there's no amount given for a vegetable, feel free to have as much as you'd like.

You will find small, frequent meals, along with a good balance of complex carbohydrates (good fiber sources) and lean protein with each meal and snack. You will notice that the fats I've suggested are the good fats that benefit your heart, such as olive oil and natural peanut butter. You won't find any sugar-sweetened drinks because I'll be moving you toward replacing those with water and other noncaloric beverages. I've also included a list of menu suggestions for meals and snacks so that your family can choose foods that sound appealing to them as well as to allow you some flexibility. For lunches, I give you options for preparing lunch at home, eating lunch at school, and eating out.

I know that we all have different tastes, so if you find that someone in your family really doesn't like a planned meal or snack of the day, feel free to choose from another day. I've included a wide variety of options, so there is something for everyone.

Most important, you'll see three categories of portion sizes under each menu suggestion. It is very straightforward: If your goal weight is 160 pounds or lower, eat the recommended portions under that category; if your goal weight is *above* 160 pounds, eat the portions recommended in that category.

For children age 12 and under, I have included a range of *suggested* portion sizes, and I emphasize that these are suggestions only. You should provide the good-quality food, and your children should determine whether they are hungry and how much they want to eat. If you exercise too much control over your children's portion sizes, it may backfire and create a potentially dangerous disordered eating situation. The suggested portion sizes can give you an idea of how much food to initially put on your child's plate. For children over age 12, follow the recommended portions for adults.

WEEK 1 MENU PLAN

◆ = goal weight 160 pounds or lower

■ = goal weight over 160 pounds

● = kids age 12 and under

▼ MONDAY

Choose one option for each meal and snack.

BREAKFAST

High-fiber, high-protein cereal with milk

◆ ½ cup cereal, 3 tablespoons protein powder, 1 cup fat-free milk

■ 1 cup cereal, 3 tablespoons protein powder, 1 cup fat-free milk

● ½ to 1 cup cereal, ½ to 1 cup low-fat milk

Low-fat cheese melted on whole grain toast

◆ 2 ounces cheese, 2 slices toast

■ 2 ounces cheese, 2 slices toast, 1 cup fat-free milk

● 1 ounce cheese, ½ or 1 slice toast

Whole Wheat Pancakes (page 239), low-fat or vegetarian sausage

◆ 2 pancakes, 2 pieces sausage

■ 3 pancakes, 3 pieces sausage

● 1 or 2 pancakes, 1 or 2 pieces sausage

SNACK

Fruit Smoothie (page 263)

◆ ½ serving smoothie

■ 1 serving smoothie, 2 tablespoons protein powder

● ¼ serving smoothie

Celery with thinly spread peanut butter topped with raisins

◆ 1 rib celery, 1 teaspoon peanut butter, 1 tablespoon raisins

■ 1 rib celery, 1 teaspoon peanut butter, 1 tablespoon raisins, 1 ounce turkey

● ½ to 1 rib celery, ½ to 1 teaspoon peanut butter, ½ to 1 tablespoon raisins

Hard-cooked egg on whole grain toast

- ◆ 1 egg, 1 slice toast

- ■ 1 egg and 1 egg white, 1 slice toast

- ● ½ egg, ½ or 1 slice toast

LUNCH (EAT IN)

Minestrone soup, small whole grain roll, side salad with olive oil vinaigrette

- ◆ 1 cup soup, 1 roll, 1 cup salad with 1 teaspoon olive oil and balsamic vinegar

- ■ 2 cups soup, 1 roll, 1 cup salad with 1 teaspoon olive oil and balsamic vinegar

- ● ½ to 1 cup soup, ½ to 1 roll, ¼ to ½ cup salad with ½ teaspoon olive oil and balsamic vinegar

LUNCH (EAT OUT)

Boston Market rotisserie chicken, sesame broccoli, sweet corn, milk

- ◆ 2 ounces chicken, broccoli, ½ cup corn, 1 cup fat-free milk

- ■ 3 ounces chicken, broccoli, 1 cup corn, 1 cup fat-free milk

- ● 1 to 3 ounces chicken, broccoli, ¼ to ½ cup corn, ½ to 1 cup low-fat milk

LUNCH (AT SCHOOL)

Zesty Tuna Salad (page 242), small whole grain roll, fruit, baby carrots

- ◆ ½ serving tuna salad, 1 roll, ½ cup fruit, carrots

- ■ ½ serving tuna salad, 1 roll, 1 cup fruit, carrots

- ● ¼ to ½ serving tuna salad, ½ to 1 roll, ½ to 1 cup fruit, carrots

SNACK

Low-fat cottage cheese with pineapple chunks

- ◆ ¼ cup cottage cheese, ½ cup pineapple

- ■ ½ cup cottage cheese, 1 cup pineapple, 8 almonds

- ● ¼ to ½ cup cottage cheese, ¼ to ½ cup pineapple

Trail mix made with Wheat Chex, peanuts or almonds, and raisins

- ◆ ¼ cup Wheat Chex, ½ tablespoon nuts, 1 tablespoon raisins

- ■ ½ cup Wheat Chex, 1 tablespoon nuts, 2 tablespoons raisins

- ● ¼ to ½ cup Wheat Chex, ½ tablespoon nuts, ½ to 1 tablespoon raisins

Low-fat vanilla yogurt, orange

- ◆ ½ cup yogurt, ½ orange

- ■ 1 cup yogurt, 1 orange

- ● ¼ to ½ cup yogurt, ¼ to ½ orange

DINNER

Lean roast pork tenderloin; whole wheat pasta sprinkled with freshly grated Parmesan cheese; Broccoli, Orange, and Watercress Salad (page 257)

- ◆ 3 ounces pork, ½ cup pasta with 1 tablespoon cheese, 1 serving salad

- ■ 4 ounces pork, ½ cup pasta with 1 tablespoon cheese, 1 serving salad

- 1 to 2 ounces pork, ¼ to ½ cup pasta with ½ to 1 tablespoon cheese, ¼ to ½ serving salad

Broiled tuna with fresh lemon, steamed broccoli, brown rice, milk

- ◆ 3 ounces tuna, broccoli, ⅓ cup rice, 1 cup fat-free milk

- ■ 4 ounces tuna, broccoli, ⅔ cup rice, 1 cup fat-free milk

- ● 1 to 2 ounces tuna, broccoli, ¼ to ⅓ cup rice, ½ to 1 cup low-fat milk

Homemade Pita Pizzas (page 245), side salad with olive oil vinaigrette, milk

- ◆ 1 pizza, 1 cup salad with 1 teaspoon olive oil and balsamic vinegar, 1 cup fat-free milk

- ■ 2 pizzas, 1 cup salad with 1 teaspoon olive oil and balsamic vinegar, 1 cup fat-free milk

- ● ½ to 1 pizza, ¼ to ½ cup salad with ½ teaspoon olive oil and balsamic vinegar, ½ to 1 cup low-fat milk

▼ TUESDAY

Choose one option for each meal and snack.

BREAKFAST

Oatmeal with milk

- ◆ ½ cup oatmeal, 1 tablespoon protein powder, 1 cup fat-free milk

- ■ 1 cup oatmeal, 2 tablespoons protein powder, 1 cup fat-free milk

- ● ½ to 1 cup oatmeal, ½ to 1 cup low-fat milk

Low-fat vanilla yogurt with fresh fruit

- ◆ 1 cup yogurt, ½ piece fruit

- ■ 1½ cups yogurt, 1 piece fruit

- ● ½ to 1 cup yogurt, ¼ to ½ piece fruit

Shrimp and Veggie Omelet (page 240) with whole grain toast

- ◆ 1 serving omelet, 1 slice toast

- ■ 1 serving omelet, 1 slice toast

- ● ¼ to ½ serving omelet, ½ to 1 slice toast

SNACK

Low-fat vanilla yogurt mixed with frozen blueberries and sunflower seeds

- ◆ ½ cup yogurt, 2 tablespoons blueberries, 2 teaspoons sunflower seeds

- ■ 1 cup yogurt, 2 tablespoons blueberries, 1 tablespoon sunflower seeds

- ● ¼ to ½ cup yogurt, 1 to 2 tablespoons blueberries, 1 teaspoon sunflower seeds

Ham sandwich on whole grain bread with tomato slices, sprinkled with lemon pepper

- ◆ 1 slice bread, 1 ounce ham, tomatoes
- ■ 1 slice bread, 2 ounces ham, tomatoes
- ● ½ to 1 slice bread, ½ to 1 ounce ham, tomatoes

Apple slices spread thinly with peanut butter

- ◆ 1 apple, 1 teaspoon peanut butter
- ■ 1 apple, 1 teaspoon peanut butter, 1 ounce turkey
- ● ¼ to ½ apple, ½ to 1 teaspoon peanut butter

LUNCH (EAT IN)

Chili made with lean ground beef, kidney beans, diced carrots, and green peppers; fresh orange sections

- ◆ 2 ounces beef; ½ cup beans, carrots, and green peppers; 1 orange
- ■ 3 ounces beef; 1 cup beans, carrots, and green peppers; 1 orange
- ● 1 to 2 ounces beef; ¼ to ½ cup beans, carrots, and green peppers; ¼ to ½ orange

LUNCH (EAT OUT)

Taco Bell bean burrito "Fresco style," orange

- ◆ ½ burrito, 1 orange
- ■ 1 burrito, 1 orange
- ● ¼ to ½ burrito, ¼ to ½ orange

LUNCH (AT SCHOOL)

Turkey sandwich on whole grain bread with lettuce and tomato, side dish of grape tomatoes, watermelon cubes

- ◆ 1 slice bread, 2 ounces turkey, lettuce and tomato, grape tomatoes, 1 cup watermelon cubes
- ■ 2 slices bread, 3 ounces turkey, lettuce and tomato, grape tomatoes, 1 cup watermelon cubes
- ● ½ to 1 slice bread, 1 ounce turkey, lettuce and tomato, grape tomatoes, ¼ to ½ cup watermelon cubes

SNACK

Low-fat Cheddar cheese with whole grain crackers, apple

- ◆ 1 ounce cheese, 3 crackers, ½ apple
- ■ 2 ounces cheese, 6 crackers, 1 apple
- ● ½ to 1 ounce cheese, 3 crackers, ¼ to ½ apple

Fresh Homemade Salsa (page 260) with baked chips

- ◆ Salsa, 6 chips
- ■ Salsa, 12 chips
- ● Salsa, 6 chips

Low-fat vanilla yogurt with sliced fresh strawberries

- ◆ ½ cup yogurt, ½ cup strawberries
- ■ 1 cup yogurt, ½ cup strawberries

- ¼ to ½ cup yogurt, ¼ to ½ cup strawberries

DINNER

Roasted skinless chicken breast, Chickpea Salad with Red Onion and Tomato (page 256), milk

- ◆ 3 ounces chicken, 1 serving salad, 1 cup fat-free milk

- ■ 4 ounces chicken, 1½ servings salad, 1 cup fat-free milk

- ● 1 to 2 ounces chicken, ¼ to ½ serving salad, ½ to 1 cup low-fat milk

Grilled Salmon (page 245), baked sweet potato, steamed broccoli and cauliflower, milk

- ◆ 1 serving salmon, 1 small sweet potato with 1 teaspoon butter, broccoli and cauliflower, 1 cup fat-free milk

- ■ 1 serving salmon, 1 large sweet potato with 1 teaspoon butter, broccoli and cauliflower, 1 cup fat-free milk

- ● ½ serving salmon, ¼ to ½ small sweet potato with ½ teaspoon butter, broccoli and cauliflower, ½ to 1 cup low-fat milk

Lean beef hamburger, Baked French Fries (page 255), steamed carrots, milk

- ◆ 3-ounce hamburger, 1 serving fries, carrots, 1 cup fat-free milk

- ■ 4-ounce hamburger, 2 servings fries, carrots, 1 cup fat-free milk

- ● 1- to 2-ounce hamburger, ¼ to ½ serving fries, carrots, ½ to 1 cup low-fat milk

▼ WEDNESDAY

Choose one option for each meal and snack.

BREAKFAST

Whole grain frozen waffles, vegetarian or low-fat sausage

- ◆ 2 waffles, 2 pieces sausage

- ■ 3 waffles, 3 pieces sausage

- ● 1 to 1½ waffles, 1 piece sausage

Fruit Smoothie (page 263)

- ◆ ½ serving smoothie

- ■ 1 serving smoothie, 2 tablespoons protein powder

- ● ¼ serving smoothie

Breakfast Sandwich (page 237)

- ◆ 1 sandwich

- ■ 1 sandwich, 1 piece fruit

- ● ½ sandwich

SNACK

Spicy Bean Dip (page 261) with small toasted whole wheat pita, fresh veggies

- ◆ ¼ cup dip, veggies, ½ pita
- ■ ¼ cup dip, veggies, 1 pita
- ● 2 tablespoons dip, veggies, ½ pita

Low-fat cottage cheese with fresh cherries

- ◆ ¼ cup cottage cheese, 6 cherries
- ■ ½ cup cottage cheese, 12 cherries
- ● 2 tablespoons cottage cheese, 4 to 6 cherries

Apple Ladybug Treats (page 260)

- ◆ 1 serving treats, 1 ounce ham
- ■ 1 serving treats, 2 ounces ham
- ● 1 serving treats

LUNCH (EAT IN)

Veggie burger on whole grain bun with lettuce and tomato, baby carrots, grapes

- ◆ 1 bun, 1 burger, lettuce and tomato, carrots, 15 grapes
- ■ 1 bun, 1 burger, lettuce and tomato, carrots, 15 grapes, 1 cup fat-free milk
- ● ½ bun, ¼ to ½ burger, lettuce and tomato, carrots, 6 to 10 grapes

LUNCH (EAT OUT)

Arby's roast beef wrap with light cheese and no sauce

- ◆ 1 wrap
- ■ 1 wrap, 1 cup fat-free milk
- ● ¼ to ½ wrap

LUNCH (AT SCHOOL)

Egg Salad (page 242) on whole grain bread, cucumber slices, red grapes

- ◆ 1 slice bread, 1 serving egg salad, cucumber slices, 15 grapes
- ■ 1 slice bread, 1 serving egg salad, cucumber slices, 15 grapes, 1 cup fat-free milk
- ● ½ to 1 slice bread, ½ serving egg salad, cucumber slices, 6 to 10 grapes

SNACK

Protein bar (14+ grams protein, 25 grams carbohydrates, less than 3 grams fat)

- ◆ ½ energy bar
- ■ 1 energy bar
- ● ¼ to ½ energy bar

Reduced-fat mozzarella sticks and fresh pear

- ◆ 1 cheese stick, 1 pear
- ■ 2 cheese sticks, 1 pear
- ● ½ cheese stick, ½ pear

Thinly spread peanut butter on whole grain toast, apple

- ◆ ½ teaspoon peanut butter, ½ slice toast, ½ apple, 1 ounce turkey

- ■ 1 teaspoon peanut butter, 1 slice toast, 1 apple, 1 ounce turkey

- ● ½ teaspoon peanut butter, ¼ to ½ slice toast, ¼ to ½ apple

DINNER

Grilled Salmon (page 245), steamed green beans, low-fat Cheddar cheese melted over brown rice mixed with steamed spinach, milk

- ◆ 1 serving salmon, green beans, ⅓ cup brown rice with spinach, 1 ounce cheese, 1 cup fat-free milk

- ■ 1 serving salmon, green beans, ⅔ cup brown rice with spinach, 1 ounce cheese, 1 cup fat-free milk

- ● ½ serving salmon, green beans, 2 to 4 tablespoons brown rice with spinach, ½ to 1 ounce cheese, ½ to 1 cup low-fat milk

Lean roast pork tenderloin, whole wheat pasta with freshly grated Parmesan cheese, side salad with olive oil vinaigrette, milk

- ◆ 3 ounces pork, ½ cup pasta with 1 tablespoon cheese, 1 cup salad with 1 teaspoon olive oil and balsamic vinegar, 1 cup fat-free milk

- ■ 4 ounces pork, 1 cup pasta with 1 tablespoon cheese, 1 cup salad with 1 teaspoon olive oil and balsamic vinegar, 1 cup fat-free milk

- ● 1 to 2 ounces pork, ¼ cup pasta with ½ tablespoon cheese, ¼ to ½ cup salad with ½ teaspoon olive oil and balsamic vinegar, ½ to 1 cup low-fat milk

Black Bean Soup (page 248); sliced tomato, fresh mozzarella, and basil salad sprinkled with balsamic vinaigrette; milk

- ◆ 1 serving soup, tomatoes with ½ ounce cheese and basil, 1 cup fat-free milk

- ■ 1 serving soup, tomatoes with 1 ounce cheese and basil, 1 cup fat-free milk

- ● ¼ to ½ serving soup, tomatoes with ½ ounce cheese and basil, ½ to 1 cup low-fat milk

▼THURSDAY

Choose one option for each meal and snack.

BREAKFAST

Breakfast Sandwich (page 237)

- ◆ 1 sandwich

- ■ 1 sandwich, 1 piece fruit

- ● ½ sandwich

Oatmeal with milk

- ◆ ½ cup oatmeal, 1 tablespoon protein powder, 1 cup fat-free milk

- ■ 1 cup oatmeal, 2 tablespoons protein powder, 1 cup fat-free milk

- ● ½ to 1 cup oatmeal, ½ to 1 cup low-fat milk

Low-fat vanilla yogurt with fresh fruit

- ◆ 1 cup yogurt, ½ piece fruit

- ■ 1½ cups yogurt, 1 piece fruit

- ● ½ to 1 cup yogurt, ¼ to ½ piece fruit

SNACK

Reduced-fat mozzarella sticks and raisins

- ◆ 1 cheese stick, 2 tablespoons raisins

- ■ 2 cheese sticks, 4 tablespoons raisins

- ● ½ to 1 cheese stick, 1 to 2 tablespoons raisins

Apple Ladybug Treats (page 260)

- ◆ 1 serving treats, 1 ounce ham

- ■ 1 serving treats, 2 ounces ham

- ● 1 serving treats

Veggie Dip (page 262) with fresh-cut vegetables

- ◆ 1 serving dip, veggies

- ■ 1 serving dip, veggies, 1 ounce turkey

- ● ½ to 1 serving dip, veggies

LUNCH (EAT IN)

Couscous with Portobello Mushrooms and Sun-Dried Tomatoes (page 241), grilled chicken

- ◆ 1 serving couscous, 2 ounces chicken

- ■ 1 serving couscous, 3 ounces chicken

- ● ¼ to ½ serving couscous, 1 to 2 ounces chicken

LUNCH (EAT OUT)

Subway turkey sandwich on 6" whole wheat wrap with 1 added fat (either cheese, oil, or mayo), grapes

- ◆ 1 wrap with 1 added fat, 15 grapes

- ■ 1 wrap with 1 added fat, 15 grapes, 1 cup fat-free milk

- ● ½ wrap with 1 added fat, 6 to 10 grapes

LUNCH (AT SCHOOL)

Roast beef sandwich on whole grain bread, side salad with olive oil vinaigrette, cantaloupe cubes

- ◆ 1 slice bread, 2 ounces roast beef, 1 cup salad with 1 teaspoon olive oil and balsamic vinegar, 1 cup cantaloupe cubes

- ■ 2 slices bread, 3 ounces roast beef, 1 cup salad with 1 teaspoon olive oil and balsamic vinegar, 1 cup cantaloupe cubes

- ● 1 slice bread, 1 to 2 ounces roast beef, ½ cup salad with ½ teaspoon olive oil and balsamic vinegar, ¼ to ½ cup cantaloupe cubes

SNACK

Edamame (soybeans)—buy fresh or frozen and boil. If precooked, heat in microwave.

- ½ cup edamame

- 1 cup edamame

- ¼ cup edamame

Turkey sandwich with fresh tomato on whole grain bread

- 1 slice bread, 1 ounce turkey, tomato slices

- 2 slices bread, 2 ounces turkey, tomato slices

- ¼ to ½ slice bread, ½ to 1 ounce turkey, tomato slices

Protein bar (14+ grams protein, 25 grams carbohydrates, less than 3 grams fat)

- ½ energy bar

- 1 energy bar

- ¼ to ½ energy bar

DINNER

Chicken or tofu stir-fry with broccoli, water chestnuts, and carrots; brown rice; milk

- 3 ounces chicken or tofu, vegetables, ⅓ cup rice, 1 cup fat-free milk

- 4 ounces chicken or tofu, vegetables, ⅔ cup rice, 1 cup fat-free milk

- 2 to 3 ounces chicken or tofu, vegetables, 2 to 4 tablespoons rice, ½ to 1 cup low-fat milk

Grilled lean steak, Roasted Vegetables (page 258), red potatoes

- 3 ounces steak, 1 serving vegetables, 1 cup potatoes

- 4 ounces steak, 1 serving vegetables, 1½ cups potatoes

- 2 to 3 ounces steak, ½ to 1 serving vegetables, ½ to 1 cup potatoes

Soft tacos made with whole wheat tortillas, lean grilled steak or chicken, tomatoes and lettuce, and low-fat cheese; milk

- 2 tortillas, 3 ounces meat, tomatoes and lettuce, 1 ounce cheese, 1 cup fat-free milk

- 3 tortillas, 4 ounces meat, tomatoes and lettuce, 1 ounce cheese, 1 cup fat-free milk

- 1 tortilla, 1 to 2 ounces meat, tomatoes and lettuce, ½ to 1 ounce cheese, ½ to 1 cup low-fat milk

Choose one option for each meal and snack.

BREAKFAST

Breakfast Sandwich (page 237)

◆ 1 sandwich

■ 1 sandwich, 1 piece fruit

● ½ sandwich

Oatmeal with milk

◆ ½ cup oatmeal, 1 tablespoon protein powder, 1 cup fat-free milk

■ 1 cup oatmeal, 2 tablespoons protein powder, 1 cup fat-free milk

● ½ to 1 cup oatmeal, ½ to 1 cup low-fat milk

Scrambled egg with whole grain toast

◆ 1 egg and 1 egg white, 2 slices toast

■ 1 egg and 2 egg whites, 3 slices toast

● 1 egg, 1 slice toast

SNACK

Fun Fruit Kebabs (page 263) dipped in low-fat vanilla yogurt

◆ 1 kebab, ½ cup yogurt

■ 1 kebab, ½ cup yogurt mixed with ¼ cup cottage cheese

● ½ to 1 kebab, ¼ to ½ cup yogurt

Apple slices spread thinly with peanut butter

◆ 1 apple, 1 teaspoon peanut butter

■ 1 apple, 1 teaspoon peanut butter, 1 ounce turkey

● ¼ to ½ apple, ½ to 1 teaspoon peanut butter

Low-fat cheese with grapes

◆ 1 ounce cheese, 15 grapes

■ 2 ounces cheese, 15 grapes

● ½ to 1 ounce cheese, 6 to 10 grapes

LUNCH (EAT IN)

Split pea soup made with ham, carrots, celery, and onions; small whole grain roll

◆ 1 cup soup (with 1 ounce ham), 1 roll

■ 1½ cups soup (with 2 ounces ham), 1 roll

● ½ to ¾ cup soup (with ½ to 1 ounce ham), ½ roll

LUNCH (EAT OUT)

Chicken vegetable soup, small whole grain roll, side salad with olive oil vinaigrette

◆ 1 cup soup (with 2 ounces chicken), 1 roll, 1 cup salad with 1 teaspoon olive oil and balsamic vinegar

■ 2 cups soup (with 3 ounces chicken), 1 roll, 1 cup salad with 1 teaspoon olive oil and balsamic vinegar

● ½ to ¾ cup soup (with 1 ounce chicken), ½ roll, ½ cup salad with ½ teaspoon olive oil and balsamic vinegar

LUNCH (AT SCHOOL)

Peanut butter and jelly sandwich on whole grain bread (with natural peanut butter and all-fruit jam), grapes

- ◆ 1 slice bread, 1 teaspoon peanut butter, 1 teaspoon jam, 15 grapes

- ■ 2 slices bread, 2 teaspoons peanut butter, 1½ teaspoons jam, 15 grapes

- ● ½ to 1 slice bread, ½ to 1 teaspoon peanut butter, 1 teaspoon jam, 6 to 10 grapes

SNACK

Turkey and low-fat cheese slices on whole grain crackers, dried apricots

- ◆ ½ ounce turkey, ½ ounce cheese, 3 crackers, 2 apricots

- ■ 1 ounce turkey, 1 ounce cheese, 6 crackers, 4 apricots

- ● ½ ounce turkey, ½ ounce cheese, 2 to 3 crackers, 1 apricot

Low-fat cottage cheese mixed with low-fat sour cream and sprinkled with cinnamon and brown sugar, with fresh fruit for dipping

- ◆ ¼ cup cottage cheese, 1 tablespoon sour cream, ½ cup fruit

- ■ ½ cup cottage cheese, 1 tablespoon sour cream, ½ cup fruit

- ● 2 to 3 tablespoons cottage cheese, ½ tablespoon sour cream, ¼ cup fruit

Fruit Smoothie (page 263)

- ◆ ½ serving smoothie

- ■ 1 serving smoothie, 2 tablespoons protein powder

- ● ¼ serving smoothie

DINNER

Grilled Beef Tenderloin (page 249), baked potato with low-fat sour cream, Roasted Asparagus (page 258), milk

- ◆ ½ serving beef, 1 small potato with 1 tablespoon sour cream, 1 serving asparagus, 1 cup fat-free milk

- ■ ½ serving beef, 1 large potato with 1 tablespoon sour cream, 1 serving asparagus, 1 cup fat-free milk

- ● ¼ serving beef, ½ small potato with ½ tablespoon sour cream, ½ serving asparagus, ½ to 1 cup low-fat milk

Roasted skinless chicken breast, red potatoes, steamed cabbage, milk

- ◆ 3 ounces chicken, ½ cup potatoes, ½ cup cabbage, 1 cup fat-free milk

- ■ 4 ounces chicken, 1 cup potatoes, ½ cup cabbage, 1 cup fat-free milk

- ● 1 to 2 ounces chicken, ¼ cup potatoes, ¼ cup cabbage, ½ to 1 cup low-fat milk

Quick and Spicy Fish Fillets (page 246), brown rice pilaf, Green Beans with Toasted Almonds (page 259), milk

- ◆ 1 serving fish, ⅓ cup pilaf, 1 serving green beans, 1 cup fat-free milk

- 1 serving fish, ⅔ cup pilaf, 1 serving green beans, 1 cup fat-free milk

- ½ serving fish, 3 to 4 tablespoons pilaf, ½ serving green beans, ½ to 1 cup low-fat milk

▼ SATURDAY

Choose one option for each meal and snack.

BREAKFAST

Spinach and Feta Omelet (page 238)

- ◆ 1 serving omelet

- ■ 1 serving omelet

- ● ¼ to ½ serving omelet

French toast made with whole grain bread, vegetarian or low-fat sausage

- ◆ 2 slices French toast, 1 piece sausage

- ■ 3 slices French toast, 2 pieces sausage

- ● ½ to 1 slice French toast, 1 piece sausage

High-fiber, high-protein cereal with milk

- ◆ ½ cup cereal, 3 tablespoons protein powder, 1 cup fat-free milk

- ■ 1 cup cereal, 3 tablespoons protein powder, 1 cup fat-free milk

- ● ½ to 1 cup cereal, ½ to 1 cup low-fat milk

SNACK

One-half peanut butter and jelly sandwich with sliced strawberries (with natural peanut butter and all-fruit jam)

- ◆ ½ slice bread, ½ teaspoon peanut butter, ½ teaspoon jam, ½ cup strawberries

- ■ 1 slice bread, 1 teaspoon peanut butter, 1 teaspoon jam, ½ cup strawberries

- ● ½ slice bread, ½ teaspoon peanut butter, ½ teaspoon jam, ¼ cup strawberries

Hummus and fresh vegetables

- ◆ 4 tablespoons hummus, vegetables

- ■ 6 tablespoons hummus, vegetables

- ● 2 tablespoons hummus, vegetables

Low-fat vanilla yogurt with orange slices

- ◆ ½ cup yogurt, ½ orange

- ■ ½ cup yogurt mixed with ¼ cup cottage cheese, ½ orange

- ● ¼ to ½ cup yogurt, ¼ orange

LUNCH (EAT IN)

Wild Rice Apple Salad (page 255), grilled chicken

- ◆ ½ serving salad, 2 ounces chicken

- ■ 1 serving salad, 3 ounces chicken

- ● ¼ serving salad, 1 ounce chicken

Whole wheat pasta and tuna, steamed carrots, milk

- ◆ ½ cup pasta, 2 ounces tuna, carrots, 1 cup fat-free milk

- ■ 1 cup pasta, 3 ounces tuna, carrots, 1 cup fat-free milk

- ● 1 to 2 ounces tuna, ¼ cup pasta, carrots, ½ to 1 cup low-fat milk

LUNCH (EAT OUT)

Grilled chicken sandwich on whole wheat bun, steamed vegetables

- ◆ 1 bun, 2 ounces chicken, vegetables

- ■ 1 bun, 3 ounces chicken, vegetables, 1 apple

- ● ½ bun, 1 to 2 ounces chicken, vegetables

SNACK

Veggie Dip (page 262), fresh-cut vegetables

- ◆ 1 serving dip, vegetables

- ■ 2 servings dip, vegetables

- ● ½ serving dip, vegetables

Zesty Tuna Salad (page 242), on whole grain crackers, apple

- ◆ ¼ serving tuna salad, 3 crackers, ½ apple

- ■ ½ serving tuna salad, 6 crackers, ½ apple

- ● ¼ serving tuna salad, 2 or 3 crackers, ¼ apple

Fresh Homemade Salsa (page 260) with baked chips

- ◆ Salsa, 6 chips

- ■ Salsa, 12 chips

- ● Salsa, 4 to 6 chips

DINNER

Homemade Pita Pizzas (page 245), side salad with olive oil vinaigrette, milk

- ◆ 1 pizza, 1 cup salad with 1 teaspoon olive oil and balsamic vinegar, 1 cup fat-free milk

- ■ 2 pizzas, 1 cup salad with 1 teaspoon olive oil and balsamic vinegar, 1 cup fat-free milk

- ● ½ to 1 pizza, ¼ to ½ cup salad with ½ teaspoon olive oil and balsamic vinegar, ½ to 1 cup low-fat milk

Feta-Stuffed Chicken (page 247), side salad with olive oil vinaigrette

- ◆ 1 serving chicken, 1 cup salad with 1 teaspoon olive oil and balsamic vinegar

- ■ 1 serving chicken, 1 cup salad with 1 teaspoon olive oil and balsamic vinegar

- ● ¼ to ½ serving chicken, ¼ to ½ cup salad with ½ teaspoon olive oil and balsamic vinegar

Baked chicken strips, Baked French Fries (page 255), steamed cauliflower sprinkled with low-fat cheese

- ◆ 3 ounces chicken, 1 serving fries, cauliflower, 1 ounce cheese

■ 4 ounces chicken, 2 servings fries, cauliflower, 1 ounce cheese

● 1 to 2 ounces chicken, ¼ to ½ serving fries, cauliflower, ½ ounce cheese

▼SUNDAY

Choose one option for each meal and snack.

BREAKFAST

Whole Wheat Pancakes (page 239), low-fat or vegetarian sausage

◆ 2 pancakes, 2 pieces sausage

■ 3 pancakes, 3 pieces sausage

● 1 or 2 pancakes, 1 or 2 pieces sausage

Ham and Vegetable Frittata (page 238) with whole grain toast

◆ 1 serving frittata, 1 slice toast

■ 1½ servings frittata, 1 slice toast

● ½ serving frittata, ½ slice toast

Oatmeal with milk

◆ ½ cup oatmeal, 1 tablespoon protein powder, 1 cup fat-free milk

■ 1 cup oatmeal, 2 tablespoons protein powder, 1 cup fat-free milk

● ½ to 1 cup oatmeal, ½ to 1 cup low-fat milk

SNACK

Low-fat cottage cheese with fresh pineapple

◆ ¼ cup cottage cheese, ½ cup pineapple

■ ½ cup cottage cheese, 1 cup pineapple

● 2 to 3 tablespoons cottage cheese, ¼ cup pineapple

Fun Fruit Kebabs (page 263) dipped in low-fat vanilla yogurt

◆ 1 kebab, ½ cup yogurt

■ 1 kebab, ½ cup yogurt mixed with ¼ cup cottage cheese

● ½ to 1 kebab, ¼ to ½ cup yogurt

Hard-cooked egg on whole grain toast

◆ 1 egg, 1 slice toast

■ 1 egg and 1 egg white, 1 slice toast

● ½ egg, ½ slice toast

LUNCH (EAT IN)

Creamy Cauliflower Soup (page 244), side salad with olive oil vinaigrette

◆ ¾ serving soup, 1 cup salad with 1 teaspoon olive oil and balsamic vinegar

■ 1 serving soup, 1 cup salad with 1 teaspoon olive oil and balsamic vinegar

● ¼ to ½ serving soup, ¼ to ½ cup salad with ½ teaspoon olive oil and balsamic vinegar

Tomato soup, whole grain crackers, baby carrots

- ◆ 1 cup soup (made with fat-free milk), 6 crackers, carrots

- ■ 1½ cups soup (made with fat-free milk), 8 crackers, carrots

- ● ½ cup soup (made with low-fat milk), 3 to 6 crackers, carrots

LUNCH (EAT OUT)

Chicken and vegetable stir-fry, brown rice

- ◆ 2 ounces chicken, vegetables, ⅔ cup rice

- ■ 3 ounces chicken, vegetables, 1 cup rice

- ● 1 to 2 ounces chicken, vegetables, 2 to 3 tablespoons rice

SNACK

Popcorn, turkey slices with fresh tomatoes sprinkled with lemon pepper

- ◆ 3 cups popcorn, 1 ounce turkey, tomatoes

- ■ 3 cups popcorn, 2 ounces turkey, tomatoes

- ● 1 cup popcorn, ½ ounce turkey, tomatoes

Celery with thinly spread peanut butter topped with raisins

- ◆ 1 rib celery, 1 teaspoon peanut butter, 1 tablespoon raisins

- ■ 1 rib celery, 1 teaspoon peanut butter, 1 tablespoon raisins, 1 ounce turkey

- ● ½ to 1 rib celery, ½ to 1 teaspoon peanut butter, ½ to 1 tablespoon raisins

Low-fat cottage cheese with fresh cherries

- ◆ ¼ cup cottage cheese, ½ cup cherries

- ■ ½ cup cottage cheese, ½ cup cherries

- ● 2 to 3 tablespoons cottage cheese, ¼ cup cherries

DINNER

Chicken Vegetable Stew (page 248), small whole grain roll, side salad with olive oil vinaigrette

- ◆ 1 serving stew, 1 roll, 1 cup salad with 1 teaspoon olive oil and balsamic vinegar

- ■ 1 serving stew, 1 roll, 1 cup salad with 1 teaspoon olive oil and balsamic vinegar

- ● ¼ to ½ serving stew, 1 roll, ¼ to ½ cup salad with ½ teaspoon olive oil and balsamic vinegar

Sloppy Joes (page 252) on whole grain bun, side salad with olive oil vinaigrette

- ◆ 1 bun, 1 serving Sloppy Joes, 1 cup salad with 1 teaspoon olive oil and balsamic vinegar

- ■ 1 bun, 1 serving Sloppy Joes, 1 cup salad with 1 teaspoon olive oil and balsamic vinegar

- ● ½ bun, ¼ to ½ serving Sloppy Joes, ¼ to ½ cup salad with ½ teaspoon olive oil and balsamic vinegar

Stuffed Peppers (page 251), small whole grain roll, side salad with grilled chicken and olive oil vinaigrette

◆ 1 serving peppers, 1 roll, 1 cup salad with 3 ounces chicken and 1 teaspoon olive oil and balsamic vinegar

■ 1 serving peppers, 1 roll, 1 cup salad with 4 ounces chicken and 1 teaspoon olive oil and balsamic vinegar

● ¼ to ½ serving peppers, 1 roll, ¼ cup salad with 1 to 2 ounces chicken and 1 teaspoon olive oil and balsamic vinegar

FITNESS FOCUS

As we go through the program, I will introduce a new form of activity each week for you and your family. This activity will be essential to you and each of your family members who wants to become healthier. Of course, all of you want to become healthier, so no spectators, just players! I recommend that someone in your family serve as the "activity coordinator" to make sure that everyone is planning and implementing their weekly activities. Ideally, you or Dad would take on this role, but it could also be a teenager. This doesn't need to be too formal; you just need someone to make sure everyone agrees on their weekly activities and goes through with them on schedule.

I will describe how to do the activity correctly and give you my recommendations for when to do it and for how long. As we go through the next few weeks, I will show you new activities to perform in addition to what you have started in previous weeks. Each kind of exercise will have guidelines for you and your spouse to follow as well as variations for different age groups of children.

Week 1: Cardiovascular Activity

Our Week 1 Fitness Focus is cardiovascular activity, which, thankfully, comes in many forms. I always tell my clients to mix it up and change things around. In other words, don't do the same thing all the time when it comes to cardiovascular exercise—unless you like only that one thing. Changing your routine keeps you from getting bored, and it continually challenges the body. It's also more fun to explore new activities.

What is a cardiovascular activity? Cardiovascular activity means that you are using your heart and lungs. You could be walking, jogging, riding a bike, hiking, or even hopping in place. In every case, your movement increases the need for oxygen, requiring your heart and lungs to do more work. You don't have to climb Mount Everest or ride a bike in the Tour de France; you just need to move more than you do when sitting or lying around the house.

My Week 1 cardiovascular recommendations are as follows.

For Adults (Age 18 and Older)

Many of us in this age group can be quite busy, no doubt. Young adults can be in school, working, or both. The rest of us may be married with children and have busy careers. Finding time for fitness can be a task all by itself! I often suggest to my clients that they find ways to combine commute times and lunch hours with a fitness activity. For instance, maybe you can bike or skateboard to and from school. Perhaps you can do it with friends, sort of like "carpooling," but with no car! If you're an older "kid" like me who can't see yourself on a skateboard, try to walk to and from work or to the train station instead of taking your car or a taxi. During your lunch hour, try walking before eating, and be sure to take the stairs more often than the elevator.

With just a little effort and creativity, you can find 20 minutes in the morning or 10 to 20 minutes throughout the day. I recommend engaging in a cardiovascular activity 4 or 5 days per week, for 20 to 30 minutes per day. Here are some examples of different cardio activities.

Walking. If you want a low-impact way to get started, this is it. Walk before you run, as they like to say!

Biking. Cycling is a lot of fun, great to do with the entire family, and great for muscle toning along with your cardio.

Tennis. The fun and competitiveness make you forget that you are getting such a great cardio workout. There are lots of neighborhood courts and many indoor facilities too.

Bowling. Stay active, have fun, and get together with friends and other couples. It's fun to join a league and play often. You do need to moderate the post-game beer and pizza to get the full benefit, though.

Jogging. Start slowly with short distances and a moderate pace. Get your heart pumping and calories burning. Go faster and longer as you get in better condition.

Golf. The swinging is great for flexibility too. Leave the cart and the caddy at the clubhouse for maximum results. Mom and Dad playing together is great, but kids can also get involved.

Cardio machines. At home or at the gym, there are so many great options, such as treadmills, elliptical machines, and lots of other different types. Follow the instructions, follow regular timed routines, and don't overdo it.

Swimming. Almost the perfect sport for cardio and endurance, not to mention all of the strength building. Best of all, it is super–low impact on your joints and muscles, so it's perfect for people who have arthritis or another condition that limits their mobility.

Kickboxing. This sport is a fun stress reducer that also builds a lot of coordination and mental focus.

Softball. Adults spend a lot of time watching their kids, but many have forgotten how much fun it is to play. Think about joining a league, or get out there with the kids on the weekend.

For Teenagers (Ages 13 to 17)

Your teenage sons and daughters may have already discovered activities they like to do. As long as they are active while doing it, you should encourage their "playtime." As your kids get older, there are many distractions that can break their active patterns and habits, so stoke the fires and keep your kids in a routine.

If your teenagers don't like to be active, you'll need to work with them to get them moving. Try something small and easy, like going for a walk with them. Ask them to help you think something through, or seek their advice. Turn this time into a bonding session by asking them about their friends or their lives. We all could do a better job of communicating with our families, so use this activity time wisely. Keep the conversation light and positive. Take these walks regularly in order to create healthy habits, especially if your child is overweight. The combination of the positive communication, the release of endorphins, and the love from a parent will wash away negative or anxious feelings that might prevent your child from being active.

For teens, I recommend 4 days per week of cardiovascular activity. They can do up to

6 days per week, but no more. Each day, teens should be active for 30 to 45 minutes. Many of the following activities can be performed outdoors or indoors.

Volleyball. Teenagers can play in the gym, at the beach, or in the backyard, in organized games or pickup games. Volleyball provides lots of agility and coordination along with the great cardio work.

Aerobics. The name says it all. It's particularly popular with girls. You'll find lots of opportunities for classes at school and the local YMCA or YWCA. Also, some health clubs have inexpensive starter or youth programs.

Dancing. Girls especially like all kinds of dancing. They can have dance parties at home or take classes. There are lots of options, such as modern dance or even Olympic-type events. Teens can even just shake it up to popular music. It's all about moving, moving, moving.

Gymnastics. Gymnastics includes great individual sports that involve coaching and supervision. Along with its cardio benefits, it's wonderful for strength and endurance. Check schools, local Ys, and clubs.

Martial arts. These provide great cardio routines and have valuable character-building, self-confidence, and self-discipline benefits.

Rowing. In the lake or on rowing machines, this fabulous cardio workout also provides great strength and endurance benefits.

Inline skating. Inline skating is an excellent cardio workout with less pounding on the joints than running. Just make sure that everyone is wearing a helmet and other protective gear.

Horseback riding. If you can find a nearby stable or club, this is a fun way for teens to stay active. Make sure there's adult supervision.

Track and field. Getting involved in organized track and field events is great for boys and girls and doesn't require specific skills or size as football and basketball do.

Water skiing. If you are lucky enough to be near water and have access to a boat, water skiing is a great active and fun sport.

For Children (Age 12 and Younger)

For both boys and girls, it is important to engage in activities that require walking, jumping, running, skipping, hopping, catching, and climbing to aid in developing their balance, agility, and coordination. Movements such as these will also allow for their natural growth spurts and patterns to occur.

I recommend a minimum of 4 days per week of cardiovascular activities. Kids should move for 30 minutes per day, and up to 7 days a week is acceptable. These activities can be done through group sports or as general play.

Baseball, soccer, basketball, touch football. These are great if your child is a "joiner" and likes organized activities. Adult supervision and coaching are excellent, though it's even better if you or your husband can help coach.

Dodgeball. This is a very fun game, but kids need to be careful.

Tag. Kids can play this old standby for hours. They have no idea how much exercise they are getting, because they are having so much fun. It's a great game if kids have lots of neighborhood friends.

Trampoline. Kids should be careful and do this only with adult supervision and with adults serving as spotters. It's a great activity for building up endurance and leg muscles.

Climbing. Find some little hills or paths out in the parks for great fun. Monkey bars are great for upper-body muscle development and keep kids entertained for hours.

Skateboarding. Skateboarding is great for the legs and cardiovascular health. Kids must always wear helmets and must go only on sidewalks—never on the street. Make sure they check for cars going in and out of driveways.

Jump rope. Jumping rope gets the heart beating and is great for leg strength. You don't need a big yard, and you can even do it indoors.

Roller skating, ice skating. Roller and ice skating are great cardio activities, and kids love them.

Bowling. Bowling builds great coordination and arm strength, and it's fun for kids and parents alike.

Martial arts. Many kids are starting martial arts at very early ages. Judo and karate are very popular and teach kids great discipline, self-control, and self-confidence.

Check your local YMCA, YWCA, and park districts for classes and events. Whatever activities you choose, supervision and proper instruction are always recommended. It's okay to ask your children what they like to do—discover what they consider to be fun. This is also a way of finding out what sports or activities they might naturally excel at. Watch out for those future Olympians! If they can't decide, feel free to suggest a daily activity and provide them with the necessary environment.

Okay, so you now know to focus on cardiovascular activities this week. You know how many times per week your family members should be moving and for how long. For the next 7 days, the "activities coordinator" should be checking in and encouraging everyone to hit their marks!

FIT FAMILY ACTIVITY

At one time during the 7 days of Week 1, I want everyone in your family to participate in one family activity for 30 minutes.

Generally, you can do whatever you want for your weekly family fun as long as it involves the entire family and is healthy, and you have a good time. But each week, I'll suggest an idea—something easy that puts the family together and begins to reinforce good habits around this weekly event.

For Week 1's Fit Family Activity, I recommend going to a park with a soccer ball and having a family soccer game. Regardless of where you live, there are plenty of park areas where you and your entire family can meet and do lots of things. If you can't find any goals, use some trashcans or plastic cones to make goals, and have a blast. Everyone loves to kick a ball.

Spend as much time as you like playing, but no less than 30 minutes. Have scoring contests with one another. See who can head the ball into the net, who can dribble the farthest, and who can kick the farthest, or have a parents versus kids game. Be creative, and you will have fun and lots of laughs. And don't forget to give yourself and your family small rewards for their healthy efforts—maybe a trip to the movie theater or some extra time staying up on the weekends. It will go a long way.

If it's raining or too cold outside, find an indoor rock climbing wall and have the whole family try to climb. Rock climbing develops hand grip and all upper body muscles, and it's a great confidence booster. Climbing on an indoor wall is safe and fun for the whole family, but be sure to have proper instruction before starting.

WEEK 1 FINAL THOUGHTS

As your family fitness coach, I want to express the importance of just getting started. Sometimes, beginning a fitness program can be tough and even seem impossible. But once you get moving, I'm sure you'll realize how good it feels to incorporate healthy foods and activity into your busy life! So let's get started together.

We've already accomplished a lot. Our meals, our fitness plans, and our family activities are all shaping up. See you next week!

WEEK 1 ACTION STEP SUMMARY

❑ Hold your Week 1 Fit Family meeting.

❑ Review your fitness profiles, goals, and strategies.

❑ Clean your cupboards; make your new grocery list.

❑ Focus on healthy breakfasts and following your new meal plans.

❑ Begin filling out your food diaries and exercise/activity journals.

❑ Start moving! Introduce cardiovascular activity into your daily routine.

❑ Get your kicks with your Fit Family Activity: soccer

❑ Schedule your Week 2 Fit Family Meeting.

Fight Fat with Your Midday Meal—At Home or Away

Welcome back. Week 1 is under your belt, so it's time to do a little evaluation of everyone's progress and efforts. First, remember to keep it in perspective: Don't expect any miracles from anyone in just 1 week. Second, expect to face a little resistance from some family members about their food consumption and exercise habits. It's natural at this stage, so don't confront it—try to understand it and then "coach" it.

For example, if your 8-year-old son is still spending too much time inside playing X-Box and not enough time going outside and playing, you should explain to him that he needs to get moving more often so he can grow to be healthy and strong. If your daughter is still drinking too much soda during the day, you must ask her to compromise a bit and have water or juice at least at breakfast and dinner. People can ease into change. What I want you to do, first and foremost, is to keep the energy and motivation high as you and your family sit down for your second Fit Family Meeting.

JUST FOR YOU, MOM

Hey, Mom—welcome to Week 2. You should be feeling great just knowing that you are healthier today than you were 7 days ago. You have become more active and have made nutritional changes that have yielded healthy weight-loss results. Remember when we talked about turning your body into a fat-burning furnace? Well, Week 2 is when you can really turn up the burners.

You will lose weight this week, Mom, if you:

❑ Do the same amount of cardiovascular exercise as last week, but just turn up your intensity a couple of notches (increases your metabolic rate).

❑ Add strength training—just one circuit (adds muscle that will burn calories—even at rest).

❑ Cut down on all sugary drinks by half (reduces carbohydrate stores, allowing fat to burn sooner).

❑ Eat all meals as early as possible in the day (metabolizes more food so that it isn't stored overnight).

With the achievable goal of losing more weight and gaining more health over the next 7 days, let's get right into Week 2!

WEEK 2 FIT FAMILY MEETING AGENDA

❑ Review food diaries and exercise/activity journals.

❑ Make adjustments through coaching and support.

❑ Discuss your meal planning and Week 2 Food Focus: lunch.

❑ Discuss and plan your Week 2 Fitness Focus: strength training.

❑ Plan your Fit Family Activity for the week: get wet.

❑ Agree on and make commitments for the next 7 days.

❑ Schedule your Week 3 Fit Family Meeting.

WEEK 2 FIT FAMILY MEETING

Your Week 2 meeting discussion should begin with recognizing the new healthy habits each family member has formed. The fact that your spouse and kids filled out food diaries and exercise/activity journals and brought them to the meeting is absolutely commendable! You and the other family members need to pat each other on the back for your Week 1 successes. This goes for the child who completed his food diary every day last week as well as the child who may have completed the journal for only a couple of days.

You want to ignite a feeling of accomplishment, so build on what each family member gives you. Remember, success breeds success, and this is an opportunity to show your support to everyone who has started to form new healthy habits. For family members who haven't made much progress, this is a time for encouragement. Your support system must always be there—in good and not-so-good times. Very much like life, isn't it?

Another wonderful result of each family member's success is the message that it sends to the rest of the group—that it *can* be done. This will inspire attitudes like "If I did it, you can do it" or "If my sister did, then I can too." As early as the start of Week 2, it is necessary to reinforce the importance of each family member's focus and commitment to reaching their goals. Use yourself or anyone else in your family who is truly engaged in the plan as an example and role model for everyone else who might need encouragement. Emulating role models in your family can be a helpful tool to keep everyone moving forward—together.

REVIEW YOUR FOOD DIARIES

Before we talk about our new food focus for this week, we want to review your family's food diaries from last week. During your Fit Family Meeting, go around the table and have each person report what was the biggest eye-opener for them during the food diary process as well as any area that gave them trouble. Some of you may earn gold stars for having perfect records that follow my meal plan to the letter. A big bravo to them! It is my experience that most people take a little longer than 1 week to implement changes, so if others haven't followed the meal plan exactly, it's okay for now.

During the review of your food records, you may discover that one or more family members have been having difficulty remembering or finding the time to record their food intake. If this is the case, use your family support team to help brainstorm solutions. Some people find it helpful to carry a small notebook with them to record what they've eaten after each meal. Some families I've worked with have found it helpful to keep the record on the fridge, and some even write down next to

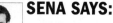

SENA SAYS:
The Week 2 meeting is a critical point to help the family work through the expected tough spots and to provide mutual support for each other.

their records what they plan to eat for the day, which I think is a great idea. Of course, you might have days that are so busy that you don't get to your diary until bedtime. It won't be as accurate, but that's still okay. The key is to find what works for you and your family so that it can become a consistent, routine part of your day.

Make Corrections

The great value of the food diary is that it gives you an opportunity to make corrections—starting now. Did you and your family members make the break from unhealthy fast foods? Did you follow the healthy breakfast recommendations from Week 1? Did you cut back on sugary drinks? The answers will be a mixed bag. The important thing is that you catch the unhealthy behaviors and replace them this week with healthy alternatives. Next week, we'll talk about the importance of monitoring your portion sizes, so keep that in mind this week as you're filling out those diaries and dishing up that food!

WEEK 2 FOOD FOCUS: HEALTHY LUNCHES

Variety is the spice of life, so let's include some new lunch options to take to school or work. It is very easy to get stuck in a rut, going through the drive-thru for a burger or packing peanut butter and jelly in the lunch box every day. I understand—I use the drive-thru occasionally and the no-brainer PB&J too. Those old standbys are fine as long as they meet your meal plan guidelines, but you may be surprised how much you enjoy trying some new foods for your midday meal. Kids sometimes have difficulty thinking "outside the lunch box" when it comes to trying new foods, so it's fine for them to venture out more slowly.

Taking lunch to work or school is really going to be your best bet for a number of reasons. For starters, it will definitely save you money. Even more important, you will have control of what is going into your body. When eating out, you lose control of how food is prepared, so even something that seems healthy on the menu may be prepared with extra fat. In addition, portion sizes can be an issue, as can the temptations of other not-so-healthy menu items and desserts. Of course, eating out is sometimes unavoidable. I'll give you two lists of lunch ideas—one for preparing food at home and one with safe bets for eating out.

Making Lunch

The sky is the limit when preparing foods, depending on how much effort and time you want to put into cooking. If you love to cook, peruse cookbooks that have a low-fat, whole-food emphasis. If you don't like to cook or don't have the time, there are plenty of quick and easy meals that can be thrown together in just a few minutes.

For lunch, sandwiches, soups, and salads tend to be quick and convenient. Sandwich fillings should be a lean lunch meat, such as turkey, chicken, roast beef, or tuna. To add variety, try different vegetables, such as cucumber slices, sprouts, or shredded carrots, or spreads such as avocado or cranberry sauce. And mix up what you put these ingredients on—you don't necessarily have to stick to bread. Try whole wheat English muffins, whole wheat pita bread, or whole wheat tortillas. You can roll up the tortillas and slice them into circles or stuff the pitas with your favorite fillings.

For lunch, I also like the ease of one-pot soups and chili. They're a great way to add vegetables to your meal plan. Follow a recipe such as beef barley or minestrone, or make up your own. Turn to the recipes in appendix A for some delicious soup ideas.

Salads can include a vegetable salad with chicken or tuna and chickpeas or have a grain base, such as brown rice with roasted vegetables or couscous with white beans. Enjoy experimenting!

Eating Out

Here are some suggestions for healthy lunches when eating at fast-food restaurants. In Week 3, I will give more tips for healthy choices at sit-down restaurants.

Boston Market. Boston Market has a great variety of low-fat vegetable side dishes such as sesame broccoli, steamed vegetable medley, sweet corn, butternut squash, and garlic-dill new potatoes. These are great when paired with their lean rotisserie chicken or turkey.

Taco Bell. I like the healthy options at Taco Bell because it is one of the few fast-food restaurants that offer menu choices that are high in fiber. In addition, you have the choice of substituting fresh salsa (called Fresco style) for cheese or sauce, which saves quite a few calories and grams of fat. Good choices include the bean burrito, burrito supreme (chicken or steak), enchirito (chicken, beef, or steak), chicken soft taco, and tostada (all made Fresco style).

Arby's. Arby's has a line of wrap sandwiches made with high-fiber, whole wheat tortilla wraps. The fat content is still quite high, so ask them to hold the sauce and go light on the cheese.

Subway. Subway has their "7 under 6" menu, which includes seven sandwiches and salads (choose low-fat salad dressing) with less than 6 grams of fat. Their "Atkins Friendly" wraps have 9 grams of fiber, but be careful, since these wraps are very high in fat! Try choosing the fillings from one of the "7 under 6" sandwiches, but use the wrap instead of the bread.

Wendy's. Wendy's has a line of salads that all sound quite delicious and healthy. In actual fact, salads are often a pitfall for healthy eating due to added cheese, bacon, fried chicken strips, and salad dressing. Wendy's Mandarin Chicken Salad with a low-fat salad dressing is probably your best bet, but skip the crispy noodles and almonds, which add 200 calories. If you'd like a sandwich for lunch, try the Ultimate Chicken Grill sandwich or a junior hamburger. A great warm lunch on a cold winter's day is a small serving of chili paired with a side salad or a plain baked potato. (Depending on your portion allotment, you may need to split the potato.)

WEEK 2 MENU PLAN

◆ = goal weight 160 pounds or lower

■ = goal weight over 160 pounds

● = kids age 12 and under

▼ MONDAY

Choose one option for each meal and snack.

BREAKFAST

Oatmeal with milk

- ◆ ½ cup oatmeal, 1 tablespoon protein powder, 1 cup fat-free milk

- ■ 1 cup oatmeal, 2 tablespoons protein powder, 1 cup fat-free milk

- ● ½ to 1 cup oatmeal, ½ to 1 cup low-fat milk

Whole grain frozen waffles, vegetarian or low-fat sausage

- ◆ 2 waffles, 2 pieces sausage

- ■ 3 waffles, 3 pieces sausage

- ● 1 waffle, 1 piece sausage

Breakfast Sandwich (page 237)

- ◆ 1 sandwich

- ■ 1 sandwich, 1 piece fruit

- ● ½ sandwich

SNACK

Veggie Dip (page 262) with fresh-cut vegetables

- ◆ 1 serving dip, veggies

- ■ 1 serving dip, veggies, 1 ounce turkey

- ● ½ to 1 serving dip, veggies

Trail mix made with Wheat Chex, raisins, and peanuts or almonds

- ◆ ¼ cup Wheat Chex, 1 tablespoon raisins, ½ tablespoon nuts

- ■ ½ cup Wheat Chex, 2 tablespoons raisins, 1 tablespoon nuts

- ● ¼ to ½ cup Wheat Chex, ½ to 1 tablespoon raisins, ½ tablespoon nuts

Reduced-fat mozzarella sticks with raisins

- ◆ 1 cheese stick, 2 tablespoons raisins

- ■ 2 cheese sticks, 4 tablespoons raisins

- ● ½ to 1 cheese stick, 1 to 2 tablespoons raisins

LUNCH (EAT IN)

Black Bean Soup (page 248), side salad with olive oil vinaigrette

- ◆ 1 serving soup, 1 cup salad with 1 teaspoon olive oil and balsamic vinegar

- ■ 1½ servings soup, 1 cup salad with 1 teaspoon olive oil and balsamic vinegar

- ● ½ serving soup, ¼ cup salad with ½ teaspoon olive oil and balsamic vinegar

LUNCH (EAT OUT)

Wendy's Mandarin chicken salad (no noodles or almonds) with low-fat French dressing

- ◆ 1 salad, 1 tablespoon dressing

- ■ 1 salad, 1 tablespoon dressing

- ● ¼ to ½ salad, ½ tablespoon dressing

LUNCH (AT SCHOOL)

Turkey Apple Sandwich (page 243), baby carrots

- ◆ ½ sandwich, carrots

- ■ 1 sandwich, carrots

- ● ¼ sandwich, carrots

SNACK

Low-fat cottage cheese with fresh pineapple

- ◆ ¼ cup cottage cheese, ½ cup pineapple

- ■ ½ cup cottage cheese, 1 cup pineapple

- ● 2 to 3 tablespoons cottage cheese, ¼ cup pineapple

Low-fat Cheddar cheese with whole grain crackers, apple

- ◆ 1 ounce cheese, 3 crackers, ½ apple

- ■ 1 ounce cheese, 6 crackers, ½ apple

- ● ½ ounce cheese, 2 or 3 crackers, ¼ apple

Spicy Bean Dip (page 261) with fresh veggies and toasted small whole wheat pita

- ◆ ¼ cup dip, veggies, ½ pita

- ■ ¼ cup dip, veggies, 1 pita

- ● 2 tablespoons dip, veggies, ½ pita

DINNER

Cajun-Spiced Chicken (page 247), steamed fresh green beans, brown rice

- ◆ 1 serving chicken, green beans, ⅓ cup rice

- ■ 1 serving chicken, green beans, ⅔ cup rice

- ● ¼ to ½ serving chicken, green beans, 2 to 4 tablespoons rice

Grilled tuna steaks, whole wheat angel hair pasta with steamed asparagus and carrots, sprinkled with freshly grated Parmesan cheese

- ◆ 3 ounces tuna, ½ cup pasta with vegetables, 1 ounce cheese

- ■ 4 ounces tuna, 1 cup pasta with vegetables, 1 ounce cheese

- ● 1 to 2 ounces tuna, ¼ cup pasta with vegetables, ½ ounce cheese

Lean beef steak, succotash, side salad with olive oil vinaigrette

- ◆ 3 ounces steak, ½ cup succotash, 1 cup salad with 1 teaspoon olive oil and balsamic vinegar

- 4 ounces steak, 1 cup succotash, 1 cup salad with 1 teaspoon olive oil and balsamic vinegar

- 1 to 2 ounces steak, ¼ cup succotash, ¼ to ½ cup salad with ½ teaspoon olive oil and balsamic vinegar

▼ TUESDAY

Choose one option for each meal and snack.

BREAKFAST

High-fiber, high-protein cereal with milk

- ◆ ½ cup cereal, 3 tablespoons protein powder, 1 cup fat-free milk

- ■ 1 cup cereal, 3 tablespoons protein powder, 1 cup fat-free milk

- ● ½ to 1 cup cereal, ½ to 1 cup low-fat milk

Low-fat vanilla yogurt with fresh fruit

- ◆ 1 cup yogurt, ½ piece fruit

- ■ 1½ cups yogurt, 1 piece fruit

- ● ½ to 1 cup yogurt, ¼ to ½ piece fruit

Spinach and Feta Omelet (page 238)

- ◆ 1 serving omelet

- ■ 1 serving omelet

- ● ¼ to ½ serving omelet

SNACK

Protein bar (14+ grams protein, 25 grams carbohydrates, less than 3 grams fat)

- ◆ ½ energy bar

- ■ 1 energy bar

- ● ¼ to ½ energy bar

Thinly spread peanut butter on whole grain toast, apple

- ◆ ½ slice toast, ½ teaspoon peanut butter, ½ apple

- ■ 1 slice toast, 1 teaspoon peanut butter, ½ apple

- ● ¼ to ½ slice toast, ½ teaspoon peanut butter, ¼ apple

Low-fat cottage cheese with fresh orange sections

- ◆ ¼ cup cottage cheese, 1 orange

- ■ ½ cup cottage cheese, 1 orange

- ● 2 to 3 tablespoons cottage cheese, ¼ to ½ orange

LUNCH (EAT IN)

Creamy Cauliflower Soup (page 244), side salad with olive oil vinaigrette

- ◆ ¾ serving soup, 1 cup salad with 1 teaspoon olive oil and balsamic vinegar

- ■ 1 serving soup, 1 cup salad with 1 teaspoon olive oil and balsamic vinegar

- ● ¼ to ½ serving soup, ¼ to ½ cup salad with ½ teaspoon olive oil and balsamic vinegar

LUNCH (EAT OUT)

McDonald's Chicken McGrill, side salad with Newman's Own low-fat balsamic vinaigrette dressing

- ◆ ½ sandwich, salad with 1 tablespoon dressing

- ■ 1 sandwich, salad with 1 tablespoon dressing

- ● ¼ to ½ sandwich, ½ salad with ½ tablespoon dressing

LUNCH (AT SCHOOL)

Egg Salad (page 242) sandwich on whole grain bread, grape tomatoes, red grapes

- ◆ 1 slice bread, 1 serving egg salad, tomatoes, 15 grapes

- ■ 2 slices bread, 1 serving egg salad, tomatoes, 15 grapes

- ● 1 slice bread, ¼ to ½ serving egg salad, tomatoes, 6 to 10 grapes

SNACK

Turkey sandwich with fresh tomato on whole grain bread

- ◆ 1 slice bread, 1 ounce turkey, tomatoes

- ■ 1 slice bread, 2 ounces turkey, tomatoes

- ● ½ slice bread, ½ ounce turkey, tomatoes

Edamame (soybeans)—buy fresh or frozen and boil. If precooked, heat in microwave.

- ◆ ½ cup edamame

- ■ 1 cup edamame

- ● ¼ cup edamame

Apple Ladybug Treats (page 260)

- ◆ 1 serving treats, 1 ounce ham

- ■ 1 serving treats, 2 ounces ham

- ● 1 serving treats

DINNER

Chicken or tofu stir-fry with broccoli, carrots, and water chestnuts; brown rice; milk

- ◆ 3 ounces chicken or tofu, vegetables, ⅓ cup rice, 1 cup fat-free milk

- ■ 4 ounces chicken or tofu, vegetables, ⅔ cup rice, 1 cup fat-free milk

- ● 1 to 2 ounces chicken or tofu, vegetables, 2 to 3 tablespoons rice, ½ to 1 cup low-fat milk

Asian Steak (page 253), brown rice

- ◆ 1 serving steak, ⅓ cup rice

- ■ 1 serving steak, ⅔ cup rice

- ● ¼ to ½ serving steak, 2 to 3 tablespoons rice

Soft tacos made with whole wheat tortillas, lean grilled steak or chicken, tomatoes and lettuce, and low-fat cheese; milk

- ◆ 2 tortillas, 3 ounces meat, tomatoes and lettuce, 1 ounce cheese, 1 cup fat-free milk

- ■ 3 tortillas, 4 ounces meat, tomatoes and lettuce, 1 ounce cheese, 1 cup fat-free milk

- ● 1 tortilla, 1 to 2 ounces meat, tomatoes and lettuce, ½ to 1 ounce cheese, ½ to 1 cup low-fat milk

Choose one option for each meal and snack.

BREAKFAST

Low-fat yogurt with orange slices

♦ 1 cup yogurt, ½ orange

■ 1½ cups yogurt, 1 orange

● ½ to 1 cup yogurt, ¼ to ½ orange

French toast made with whole grain bread, low-fat or vegetarian sausage

♦ 2 pieces French toast, 1 piece sausage

■ 3 pieces French toast, 2 pieces sausage

● ½ to 1 piece French toast, 1 piece sausage

Shrimp and Veggie Omelet (page 240) with whole grain toast

♦ 1 serving omelet, 1 slice toast

■ 1 serving omelet, 1 slice toast

● ¼ to ½ serving omelet, ½ to 1 slice toast

SNACK

Fruit Smoothie (page 263)

♦ ½ serving smoothie

■ 1 serving smoothie, 2 tablespoons protein powder

● ¼ serving smoothie

Low-fat cottage cheese with fresh cherries

♦ ¼ cup cottage cheese, ½ cup cherries

■ ½ cup cottage cheese, ½ cup cherries

● 2 to 3 tablespoons cottage cheese, ¼ cup cherries

Celery with thinly spread peanut butter topped with raisins

♦ 1 rib celery, 1 teaspoon peanut butter, 1 tablespoon raisins

■ 1 rib celery, 1 teaspoon peanut butter, 1 tablespoon raisins, 1 ounce turkey

● ½ to 1 rib celery, ½ to 1 teaspoon peanut butter, ½ to 1 tablespoon raisins

LUNCH (EAT IN)

Chicken Vegetable Stew (page 248), small whole grain roll, side salad with olive oil vinaigrette

♦ 1 serving stew, 1 roll, 1 cup salad with 1 teaspoon olive oil and balsamic vinegar

■ 1 serving stew, 1 roll, 1 cup salad with 1 teaspoon olive oil and balsamic vinegar

● ¼ to ½ serving stew, 1 roll, ¼ to ½ cup salad with ½ teaspoon olive oil and balsamic vinegar

LUNCH (EAT OUT)

Arby's turkey wrap sandwich with no sauce, side salad with low-fat dressing

♦ ½ sandwich, salad with 1 tablespoon dressing

■ 1 sandwich, salad with 1 tablespoon dressing

- ¼ to ½ sandwich, ¼ to ½ salad with ½ tablespoon dressing

LUNCH (AT SCHOOL)

Turkey wrap with lettuce, tomato, and cucumber slices in whole wheat tortilla (can use low-fat ranch dressing on the side), orange slices

- ◆ 1 tortilla, 2 ounces turkey, lettuce, tomato, cucumber slices, 2 tablespoons dressing, ½ orange

- ■ 2 tortillas, 3 ounces turkey, lettuce, tomato, cucumber slices, 2 tablespoons dressing, ½ orange

- ● ½ tortilla, 1 to 2 ounces turkey, lettuce, tomato, cucumber slices, 1 tablespoon dressing, ¼ to ½ orange

SNACK

Fun Fruit Kebabs (page 263) dipped in low-fat vanilla yogurt

- ◆ 1 kebab, ½ cup yogurt

- ■ 1 kebab, ½ cup yogurt mixed with ¼ cup cottage cheese

- ● ½ to 1 kebab, ¼ to ½ cup yogurt

Turkey and low-fat cheese slices on whole grain crackers, dried apricots

- ◆ ½ ounce turkey, ½ ounce cheese, 3 crackers, 2 apricots

- ■ 1 ounce turkey, 1 ounce cheese, 6 crackers, 4 apricots

- ● ½ ounce turkey, ½ ounce cheese, 2 or 3 crackers, 1 apricot

Hummus and fresh vegetables

- ◆ 4 tablespoons hummus, vegetables

- ■ 6 tablespoons hummus, vegetables

- ● 2 tablespoons hummus, vegetables

DINNER

Lean roast pork tenderloin with apple slices, steamed broccoli and cauliflower

- ◆ 3 ounces pork, 1 apple, broccoli and cauliflower

- ■ 4 ounces pork, 1 apple, 1 small roll, broccoli and cauliflower

- ● 1 to 2 ounces pork, ¼ to ½ apple, broccoli and cauliflower

Baked Fish with Vegetables (page 250), whole wheat rotini with freshly grated Parmesan cheese

- ◆ 1 serving fish with vegetables, ½ cup rotini, 1 ounce cheese

- ■ 1 serving fish with vegetables, 1 cup rotini, 1 ounce cheese

- ● ½ serving fish with vegetables, ¼ cup rotini, ½ to 1 ounce cheese

Homemade Pita Pizzas (page 245), side salad with olive oil vinaigrette, milk

- ◆ 1 pizza, 1 cup salad with 1 teaspoon olive oil and balsamic vinegar, 1 cup fat-free milk

■ 2 pizzas, 1 cup salad with 1 teaspoon olive oil and balsamic vinegar, 1 cup fat-free milk

● ½ to 1 pizza, ¼ to ½ cup salad with ½ teaspoon olive oil and balsamic vinegar, ½ to 1 cup low-fat milk

▼ THURSDAY

Choose one option for each meal and snack.

BREAKFAST

Oatmeal with milk

◆ ½ cup oatmeal, 1 tablespoon protein powder, 1 cup fat-free milk

■ 1 cup oatmeal, 2 tablespoons protein powder, 1 cup fat-free milk

● ½ to 1 cup oatmeal, ½ to 1 cup low-fat milk

Whole grain frozen waffles, vegetarian or low-fat sausage

◆ 2 waffles, 2 pieces sausage

■ 3 waffles, 3 pieces sausage

● 1 to 1½ waffles, 1 piece sausage

Low-fat cheese melted on whole grain toast

◆ 2 ounces cheese, 2 slices toast

■ 2 ounces cheese, 2 slices toast, 1 cup fat-free milk

● 1 ounce cheese, ½ to 1 slice toast

SNACK

Trail mix made with Wheat Chex, raisins, and peanuts or almonds

◆ ¼ cup Wheat Chex, 1 tablespoon raisins, ½ tablespoon nuts

■ ½ cup Wheat Chex, 2 tablespoons raisins, 1 tablespoon nuts

● ¼ to ½ cup Wheat Chex, ½ to 1 tablespoon raisins, ½ tablespoon nuts

Reduced-fat mozzarella sticks and raisins

◆ 1 cheese stick, 2 tablespoons raisins

■ 2 cheese sticks, 4 tablespoons raisins

● ½ to 1 cheese stick, 1 to 2 tablespoons raisins

Low-fat cottage cheese with fresh pineapple

◆ ¼ cup cottage cheese, ½ cup pineapple

■ ½ cup cottage cheese, 1 cup pineapple

● 2 to 3 tablespoons cottage cheese, ¼ cup pineapple

LUNCH (EAT IN)

Wild Rice Apple Salad (page 255), grilled chicken

◆ ½ serving salad, 2 ounces chicken

■ 1 serving salad, 3 ounces chicken

● ¼ serving salad, 1 ounce chicken

LUNCH (EAT OUT)

Taco Bell steak burrito supreme "Fresco style"

- ◆ 1 burrito

- ▪ 1 burrito

- ● ¼ to ½ burrito

LUNCH (AT SCHOOL)

Low-fat cheese, turkey, and tomato sandwich on whole wheat pita with Dijon mustard; apple slices; baby carrots

- ◆ 1 pita, 1 ounce cheese, 1 ounce turkey, tomato, 1 apple, carrots

- ▪ 1½ pitas, 1 ounce cheese, 2 ounces turkey, tomato, 1 apple, carrots

- ● ½ pita, ½ ounce cheese, ½ to 1 ounce turkey, tomato, ¼ to ½ apple, carrots

SNACK

Veggie Dip (page 262) with fresh-cut vegetables

- ◆ 1 serving dip, vegetables

- ▪ 2 servings dip, vegetables

- ● ½ serving dip, vegetables

Low-fat cottage cheese mixed with low-fat sour cream and sprinkled with cinnamon and brown sugar, with fresh fruit for dipping

- ◆ ¼ cup cottage cheese, 1 tablespoon sour cream, ½ cup fruit

- ▪ ½ cup cottage cheese, 1 tablespoon sour cream, ½ cup fruit

- ● 2 to 3 tablespoons cottage cheese, ½ tablespoon sour cream, ¼ cup fruit

Protein bar (14+ grams protein, 25 grams carbohydrates, less than 3 grams fat)

- ◆ ½ energy bar

- ▪ 1 energy bar

- ● ¼ to ½ energy bar

DINNER

Veggie burger on whole grain bun, Baked French Fries made with sweet potatoes (page 255), broccoli sprinkled with low-fat cheese

- ◆ 1 bun, 1 burger, 1 serving fries, broccoli with 1 ounce cheese

- ▪ 1 bun, 1 burger, 2 servings fries, broccoli with 1 ounce cheese

- ● ¼ to ½ bun, ¼ to ½ burger, ½ serving fries, broccoli with ½ to 1 ounce cheese

Grilled Salmon (page 245), Sweet Carrot Salad (page 257), Wild Rice Casserole (page 254)

- ◆ 1 serving salmon, 1 serving salad, 1 serving casserole

- ▪ 1 serving salmon, 1½ servings salad, 1½ servings casserole

- ● ½ serving salmon, ¼ to ½ serving salad, ¼ to ½ serving casserole

Cabbage Roll-Ups (page 249), side salad with olive oil vinaigrette

- ◆ 1 serving roll-ups, 1 cup salad with 1 teaspoon olive oil and balsamic vinegar

- 1½ servings roll-ups, 1 cup salad with 1 teaspoon olive oil and balsamic vinegar

- ¼ to ½ serving roll-ups, ¼ to ½ cup salad with ½ teaspoon olive oil and balsamic vinegar

▼ FRIDAY

Choose one option for each meal and snack.

BREAKFAST

High-fiber, high-protein cereal with milk

- ◆ ½ cup cereal, 3 tablespoons protein powder, 1 cup fat-free milk

- ■ 1 cup cereal, 3 tablespoons protein powder, 1 cup fat-free milk

- ● ½ to 1 cup cereal, ½ to 1 cup low-fat milk

Low-fat vanilla yogurt with sliced strawberries

- ◆ 1 cup yogurt, ½ cup strawberries

- ■ 1½ cups yogurt, 1 cup strawberries

- ● ½ to 1 cup yogurt, ¼ cup strawberries

Scrambled egg with whole grain toast

- ◆ 1 egg and 1 egg white, 2 slices toast

- ■ 1 egg and 2 egg whites, 3 slices toast

- ● 1 egg, 1 slice toast

SNACK

Spiced Pumpkin Seeds (page 262) and raisins

- ◆ ¼ cup pumpkin seeds, 1 tablespoon raisins

- ■ ¼ cup pumpkin seeds, 3 tablespoons raisins

- ● 2 to 3 tablespoons pumpkin seeds, 1 to 2 tablespoons raisins

Apple slices spread thinly with peanut butter

- ◆ 1 apple, 2 teaspoons peanut butter

- ■ 1 apple, 2 teaspoons peanut butter

- ● ¼ to ½ apple, 1 teaspoon peanut butter

Hummus with fresh vegetables

- ◆ 4 tablespoons hummus, vegetables

- ■ 6 tablespoons hummus, vegetables

- ● 2 tablespoons hummus, vegetables

LUNCH (EAT IN)

Chickpea Salad with Red Onion and Tomato (page 256) with tuna

- ◆ 1 serving salad, 2 ounces tuna

- ■ 1½ servings salad, 3 ounces tuna

- ● ¼ to ½ serving salad, 1 to 2 ounces tuna

LUNCH (EAT OUT)

Subway ham sandwich wrap

- ◆ 1 wrap

- ■ 1 wrap

- ● ¼ to ½ wrap

LUNCH (AT SCHOOL)

Vegetable Sandwich (page 243), milk

- ◆ 1 sandwich, 1 cup fat-free milk

- ■ 1 sandwich, 1 cup fat-free milk

- ● ¼ to ½ sandwich, ½ to 1 cup low-fat milk

SNACK

Fresh Homemade Salsa (page 260) with baked chips

- ◆ Salsa, 6 chips

- ■ Salsa, 12 chips

- ● Salsa, 6 chips

Edamame (soybeans)—buy fresh or frozen and boil. If precooked, heat in microwave.

- ◆ ½ cup edamame

- ■ 1 cup edamame

- ● ¼ cup edamame

Zesty Tuna Salad (page 242) on whole grain crackers, apple

- ◆ ¼ serving tuna salad, 3 crackers, ½ apple

- ■ ½ serving tuna salad, 6 crackers, ½ apple

- ● ¼ serving tuna salad, 2 or 3 crackers, ¼ apple

DINNER

Lean beef hamburger on whole grain bun, Coleslaw Salad (page 259), milk

- ◆ 1 bun, 3-ounce hamburger, 1 serving coleslaw, 1 cup fat-free milk

- ■ 1 bun, 4-ounce hamburger, 1½ servings coleslaw, 1 cup fat-free milk

- ● ½ bun, 1- to 2-ounce hamburger, ½ serving coleslaw, ½ to 1 cup low-fat milk

Homemade Pita Pizzas (page 245), side salad with olive oil vinaigrette, milk

- ◆ 1 pizza, 1 cup salad with 1 teaspoon olive oil and balsamic vinegar, 1 cup fat-free milk

- ■ 2 pizzas, 1 cup salad with 1 teaspoon olive oil and balsamic vinegar, 1 cup fat-free milk

- ● ½ to 1 pizza, ¼ to ½ cup salad with ½ teaspoon olive oil and balsamic vinegar, ½ to 1 cup low-fat milk

Cajun-Spiced Chicken (page 247), brown rice, steamed green beans, milk

- ◆ 1 serving chicken, ⅓ cup rice, green beans, 1 cup fat-free milk

- ■ 1 serving chicken, ⅔ cup rice, green beans, 1 cup fat-free milk

- ● ¼ to ½ serving chicken, 2 to 4 tablespoons rice, green beans, ½ to 1 cup low-fat milk

Choose one option for each meal and snack.

BREAKFAST

Whole Wheat Pancakes (page 239), low-fat or vegetarian sausage

- ◆ 2 pancakes, 2 pieces sausage

- ■ 3 pancakes, 3 pieces sausage

- ● 1 or 2 pancakes, 1 or 2 pieces sausage

Ham and Vegetable Frittata (page 238) with whole grain toast

- ◆ 1 serving frittata, 1 slice toast

- ■ 1½ servings frittata, 1 slice toast

- ● ½ serving frittata, ½ slice toast

Oatmeal with milk

- ◆ ½ cup oatmeal, 1 tablespoon protein powder. 1 cup fat-free milk

- ■ 1 cup oatmeal, 2 tablespoons protein powder, 1 cup fat-free milk

- ● ½ to 1 cup oatmeal, ½ to 1 cup low-fat milk

SNACK

Spinach and Artichoke Heart Dip (page 261) with small baked whole wheat pita

- ◆ 1 serving dip, 1 pita

- ■ 1½ servings dip, 1 pita

- ● ½ to 1 serving dip, ½ to 1 pita

Fun Fruit Kebabs (page 263) dipped in low-fat vanilla yogurt

- ◆ 1 kebab, ½ cup yogurt

- ■ 1 kebab, ½ cup yogurt mixed with ¼ cup cottage cheese

- ● ½ to 1 kebab, ¼ to ½ cup yogurt

Popcorn, turkey slices with fresh tomatoes sprinkled with lemon pepper

- ◆ 3 cups popcorn, 1 ounce turkey, tomatoes

- ■ 3 cups popcorn, 2 ounces turkey, tomatoes

- ● 1 cup popcorn, ½ ounce turkey, tomatoes

LUNCH (EAT IN)

Sweet Potato Minestrone (page 246), grilled chicken

- ◆ 1 serving soup, 2 ounces chicken

- ■ 1 serving soup, 3 ounces chicken

- ● ½ serving soup, 1 to 2 ounces chicken

Zesty Tuna Salad (page 242) over whole wheat angel hair pasta, small apple

- ◆ ½ serving tuna salad, ½ cup pasta, 1 apple

- ■ ½ serving tuna salad, 1 cup pasta, 1 apple

● ¼ to ½ serving tuna salad, ¼ to ½ cup pasta, ½ apple

LUNCH (EAT OUT)

Taco Bell chicken enchirito "Fresco style"

◆ 1 enchirito

■ 1 enchirito

● ¼ to ½ enchirito

SNACK

Hard-cooked egg on whole grain toast

◆ 1 egg, 1 slice toast

■ 1 egg and 1 egg white, 1 slice toast

● ½ egg, ½ slice toast

Celery with thinly spread peanut butter topped with raisins

◆ 1 rib celery, 1 teaspoon peanut butter, 1 tablespoon raisins

■ 1 rib celery, 1 teaspoon peanut butter, 1 tablespoon raisins, 1 ounce turkey

● ½ to 1 rib celery, ½ to 1 teaspoon peanut butter, ½ to 1 tablespoon raisins

Low-fat cottage cheese with fresh cherries

◆ ¼ cup cottage cheese, ½ cup cherries

■ ½ cup cottage cheese, ½ cup cherries

● 2 to 3 tablespoons cottage cheese, ¼ cup cherries

DINNER

Grilled Beef Tenderloin (page 249), baked potato with low-fat sour cream, Roasted Asparagus (page 258), milk

◆ ½ serving beef, 1 small potato, 1 tablespoon sour cream, 1 serving asparagus, 1 cup fat-free milk

■ ½ serving beef, 1 large potato, 1 tablespoon sour cream, 1 serving asparagus, 1 cup fat-free milk

● ¼ serving beef, ½ small potato, ½ tablespoon sour cream, ½ serving asparagus, ½ to 1 cup low-fat milk

Soft tacos made with whole wheat tortillas, grilled steak or chicken, tomatoes and lettuce, and low-fat cheese; milk

◆ 2 tortillas, 3 ounces meat, tomatoes and lettuce, 1 ounce cheese, 1 cup fat-free milk

■ 3 tortillas, 4 ounces meat, tomatoes and lettuce, 1 ounce cheese, 1 cup fat-free milk

● 1 tortilla, 1 to 2 ounces meat, tomatoes and lettuce, ½ to 1 ounce cheese, ½ to 1 cup low-fat milk

Sloppy Joes (page 252) on whole grain bun, Baked French Fries (page 255), steamed carrots

◆ 1 bun, 1 serving Sloppy Joes, 1 serving fries, carrots

■ 1 bun, 1 serving Sloppy Joes, 1½ servings fries, carrots

● ½ bun, ¼ to ½ serving Sloppy Joes, ½ serving fries, carrots

Choose one option for each meal and snack.

BREAKFAST

Shrimp and Veggie Omelet (page 240) with whole grain toast

- ◆ 1 serving omelet, 1 slice toast

- ■ 1 serving omelet, 1 slice toast

- ● ¼ to ½ serving omelet, ½ to 1 slice toast

French toast made with whole grain bread, low-fat or vegetarian sausage

- ◆ 2 slices French toast, 1 piece sausage

- ■ 3 slices French toast, 2 pieces sausage

- ● ½ to 1 slice French toast, 1 piece sausage

Oatmeal with milk

- ◆ ½ cup oatmeal, 1 tablespoon protein powder, 1 cup fat-free milk

- ■ 1 cup oatmeal, 2 tablespoons protein powder, 1 cup fat-free milk

- ● ½ to 1 cup oatmeal, ½ to 1 cup low-fat milk

SNACK

One-half peanut butter and jelly sandwich on whole grain bread with sliced strawberries (with natural peanut butter and all-fruit jam)

- ◆ ½ slice bread, ½ teaspoon peanut butter, ½ teaspoon jam, ½ cup strawberries

- ■ 1 slice bread, 1 teaspoon peanut butter, 1 teaspoon jam, ½ cup strawberries

- ● ½ slice bread, ½ teaspoon peanut butter, ½ teaspoon jam, ¼ cup strawberries

Apple Ladybug Treats (page 260)

- ◆ 1 serving treats, 1 ounce ham

- ■ 1 serving treats, 2 ounces ham

- ● 1 serving treats

Reduced-fat mozzarella sticks and fresh pear

- ◆ 1 cheese stick, 1 pear

- ■ 2 cheese sticks, 1 pear

- ● ½ cheese stick, ½ pear

LUNCH (EAT IN)

Chicken Salad (page 244) on whole grain bread, red grapes

- ◆ 1 slice bread, 1 serving chicken salad, 15 grapes

- ■ 1 slice bread, 1 serving chicken salad, 15 grapes

- ● ½ to 1 slice bread, ¼ to ½ serving chicken salad, 6 to 10 grapes

Roast beef sandwich on whole grain bread, side salad with olive oil vinaigrette, cantaloupe cubes

- ◆ 1 slice bread, 2 ounces roast beef, 1 cup salad with 1 teaspoon olive oil and balsamic vinegar, 1 cup cantaloupe cubes

- 2 slices bread, 3 ounces roast beef, 1 cup salad with 1 teaspoon olive oil and balsamic vinegar, 1 cup cantaloupe cubes

- ½ to 1 slice bread, 1 to 2 ounces roast beef, ¼ to ½ cup salad with ½ to 1 teaspoon olive oil and balsamic vinegar, ¼ to ½ cup cantaloupe cubes

LUNCH (EAT OUT)

Boston Market rotisserie turkey, steamed vegetable medley, butternut squash

- 2 ounces turkey, 1 cup vegetables, ½ cup squash

- 3 ounces turkey, 1 cup vegetables, 1 cup squash

- 1 to 2 ounces turkey, ¼ to ½ cup vegetables, ¼ cup squash

SNACK

Low-fat vanilla yogurt mixed with frozen blueberries and sprinkled with sunflower seeds

- ½ cup yogurt, ½ cup blueberries, 1 tablespoon sunflower seeds

- 1 cup yogurt, ½ cup blueberries, 1 tablespoon sunflower seeds

- ¼ to ½ cup yogurt, ¼ to ½ cup blueberries, 1 teaspoon sunflower seeds

Fruit Smoothie (page 263)

- ½ serving smoothie

- 1 serving smoothie, 2 tablespoons protein powder

- ¼ serving smoothie

Trail mix made with Wheat Chex, raisins, and peanuts or almonds

- ¼ cup Wheat Chex, 1 tablespoon raisins, ½ tablespoon nuts

- ½ cup Wheat Chex, 2 tablespoons raisins, 1 tablespoon nuts

- ¼ to ½ cup Wheat Chex, ½ to 1 tablespoon raisins, ½ tablespoon nuts

DINNER

Chicken Creole (page 250), side salad with olive oil vinaigrette, milk

- 1 serving creole, 1 cup salad with 1 teaspoon olive oil and balsamic vinegar, 1 cup fat-free milk

- 1 serving creole, 1 cup salad with 1 teaspoon olive oil and balsamic vinegar, 1 cup fat-free milk

- ¼ to ½ serving creole, ¼ to ½ cup salad with ½ to 1 teaspoon olive oil and balsamic vinegar, ½ to 1 cup low-fat milk

Baked Fish with Vegetables (page 250), whole wheat rotini with freshly grated Parmesan cheese

- 1 serving fish with vegetables, ½ cup rotini, 1 ounce cheese

- 1 serving fish with vegetables, 1 cup rotini, 1 ounce cheese

- ½ serving fish with vegetables, ¼ cup rotini, ½ to 1 ounce cheese

Grilled lean steak, Roasted Vegetables (page 258), red potatoes

- ◆ 3 ounces steak, 1 serving vegetables, 1 cup potatoes

- ■ 4 ounces steak, 1 serving vegetables, 1½ cups potatoes

- ● 2 to 3 ounces steak, ½ to 1 serving vegetables, ½ to 1 cup potatoes

FITNESS FOCUS

Now that we have our healthy menus in place for Week 2, it's time to turn our attention to our fitness activities. Remember, each week I'll introduce a new activity that you and your family can easily add to your schedules. Continue the activities from Week 1 that are already giving you feelings of success and just add several minutes of the new activity. As each week passes, it will get easier—and you'll get accustomed to seeing positive results!

SENA SAYS:

If your family doesn't meet short-term goals, remind them that a sports team can fall short of its short-term goal and lose the first games of the playoffs, but it can still reach its long-term goal (winning a championship)—just as the Red Sox did against my beloved Yankees in the 2004 ACLS!

Before we start on our Week 2 Fitness Focus, let's take a moment to review our exercise/activity journals from Week 1.

Review Your Exercise/Activity Journals

You'll want to review your exercise/activity journal just as you did with your food diary. At the start, don't expect your family members (or yourself) to be perfect. Instead, look for the start of healthy habits. With exercise, people tend to start out strong and then fizzle out. Your job is to buck that trend and focus on keeping to a consistent program.

After Week 1, you and your family are looking for small successes that are aligned with your goals and, most important, your strategies.

Goals

Long term: Lose 20 to 40 pounds

Short term: Lose 2 to 5 pounds per week

Strategy

Do cardiovascular exercise 3 days per week—Monday, Wednesday, and Friday—for 20 minutes per day.

Do strength training 2 days per week—Tuesday and Thursday.

What I want you to look for is the effort and commitment to follow through. The primary purpose of Weeks 1 and 2 is to establish these healthy habits as soon as possible. Let me give you an example. This is Mary's exercise/activity journal.

DAY/DATE	CARDIOVASCULAR EXERCISE (duration)	STRENGTH TRAINING (duration)
Monday 6/14	10 min	
Tuesday 6/15		15 min
Wednesday 6/16	15 min	
Thursday 6/17	Went for a 20-min walk	10 min
Friday 6/18	10 min	
Saturday		
Sunday		

Great! This looks like Mary made the effort to become more active than she was before and, by all indications, began forming some healthy habits. She wasn't perfect (she didn't put in exactly the amount of time she had planned), but the important thing is that Mary showed up. This type of progress toward goals is great, and as I mentioned before, should be recognized and supported by all family members.

Here's what a not-so-good fitness journal looks like. Although Tommy's effort was made and should be recognized by the group, he'll need some coaching.

Goals

Long term: Lose 10 to 15 pounds; make basketball team next year

Short term: Lose 1 or 2 pounds per week; become a better foul shooter

Strategy

Go for bike rides three times per week (20 minutes)

Practice foul shots two times per week (100 shots)

DAY/DATE	CARDIOVASCULAR EXERCISE (duration)	STRENGTH TRAINING (duration)
Monday 6/14	Rode bike 10 min Took 50 foul shots	
Tuesday		
Wednesday		
Thursday		
Friday		

First, we need to find out why Tommy was unable to carry out his weekly strategies, since he exercised only 1 day that week. Then we need to help him understand how important it is to do the little things that will ultimately make him feel better and enable him to reach his goal—to make the basketball team next year. You could explain to him that players like Michael Jordan and Larry Bird always worked on their foul shots, and that's how they became great. You also might want to ask Tommy what got in his way. Why didn't he show up? Did the task seem too difficult to him? If so, you can revise his goals. Reevaluating goals and revising strategies is always possible. On the other hand, Tommy could have been distracted by difficulties with his math homework. In that case, you'll have to get him some help in that area. The most important thing is that Tommy shows up, so try to find out what prevented that and adapt accordingly.

Week 2: Strength Training

Our Week 2 focus is on strength training, also known as resistance training. Strength training is any type of exercise that is weight bearing on the muscles and joints.

You can use any one type—or combination of types—of equipment, including free weights, weight machines, medicine balls, dumbbells, or rubber tubing. In any case, all of these forms of strength training will enable the body's muscles to build up and become toned, healthy, youthful, calorie-burning muscles. There's nothing like it!

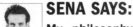

SENA SAYS:
My philosophy has always been that everyone should build strength-training exercise into their life. In my opinion, it is the fountain of youth!

Don't worry, Mom—you're not going to build big, bulky muscles just by exercising with a pair of dumbbells. By following my recommendations, though, you and your family will develop bodies that are fat-fighting machines.

Equipment to Use

There are several low-cost, professional-grade pieces of strength-training equipment that you and your family can use safely and effectively to reach all of your desired fitness goals.

Dumbbells, medicine balls, rubber tubes, and stability balls are all items that can be easily found at most sporting goods stores and other retailers that sell fitness equipment. They can also be found online under the category "fitness equipment" and in many mail-order catalogs that carry health and fitness products.

These same fitness products are "trainer's choice" when it comes to getting results. They're used by thousands of gym-goers around the country. I like these fitness tools because, first and foremost, they help my clients get the results they need. Everyone in the family can use them, and they don't take up a lot of space because they can be easily stored away under a bed, in a closet, or in a storage container in a cabinet.

General Costs

Dumbbells are usually priced by the pound—about 50 cents per pound. The total price will vary depending on the total weight. One pair of 10-pound dumbbells is approximately $10 to $12.

Medicine balls are a little more expensive, but the bigger they are, the less they cost per pound. A 6-pound ball is approximately $30; a 12-pound ball is approximately $45.

Stability balls (a.k.a. Swiss balls) can range in price from $24 to $35. Before buying or using a stability ball, each person should be measured for proper "fit." When you're sitting on top of the ball, your thighs should be level and parallel to the ground.

Rubber tubes, depending on the manufacturer, come in a variety of colors to designate the different resistance levels. Each color is priced roughly the same, ranging anywhere from $8 to $14 per tube.

HOW TO USE A DOOR ANCHOR FOR RUBBER TUBES

All door anchors are not created equal, so be sure that you buy a tube anchor that inserts into the jamb of the door rather than around the doorknob—which can be dangerous. Safety is key here!

Open the door from the inside of the room or the back side of the door whenever possible. Insert the anchor at the height specified for the exercise, then close the door completely, making sure you hear it latch. Lock the door and tug on the anchor to make sure it's secure, then insert your tube for exercising. Never use a bifold door or a door that does not have a secure frame.

Of the four fitness products mentioned above, my favorite is the rubber tube. I like it for me, my clients, and your family because of its "variable resistance." This means that as a rubber tube stretches to longer lengths, it becomes more challenging, then is less challenging as it returns to its original length. This equates to very little strain on muscles, tendons, and joints. Rubber tubes are great for the whole family. For more information on low-cost fitness solutions and more motivational tips, check out www.michaelsena.com.

How Hard Should You Be Exercising?

Use this professional scale, known as the rate of perceived exertion scale, or R.P.E. scale.

1 — 2 — 3 — 4 — 5 — 6 — 7 — 8 — 9 — 10

Not very challenging   **Somewhat challenging**   **Very challenging**

You always want to exercise in a safe range—a range that feels comfortable to you. It is true that the higher the number, the more intensity you will create. However, you must always rely on your own inner judgment to know if you are working out too hard, not hard enough, or just right. The correct intensity level is what feels like a comfortable challenge to your system. You shouldn't be gasping for air or feeling faint, light-headed, or dizzy at any time.

For beginners, I would recommend working for an intensity between 4 and 6, and for intermediate to advanced levels, 6 to 8. Always use your best judgment to prevent any serious injury.

Here are my Week 2 strength-training recommendations for safety and results—for you and your family members.

For Adults (Age 18 and Older)

It's your turn, Mom, and see if you can get your hubby to join in too. Your strength-training program is also appropriate for teenagers (ages 13 to 17). It's simple, it works all of the major muscle groups, and it's quick and balanced. These exercises can be performed in a gym or in your home.

The instructions on the following pages will walk you through one complete strength-training circuit. Even though Mom is shown doing these exercises, they're great for men too.

I recommend 3 days of strength-training exercise per week, doing one set of each exercise. Follow the number sequence to complete one go-round, or "circuit." Do 10 repetitions per exercise. Simply follow the sequence of numbers from 1 to 8 to complete a full exercise session.

Always practice good form—never forfeit form for another repetition. Remember to consult your physician before performing this or any other exercise program.

#1 CHEST PRESS
(CHEST, SHOULDERS, TRICEPS)

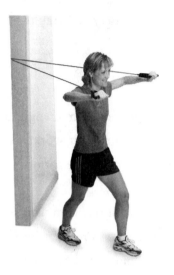 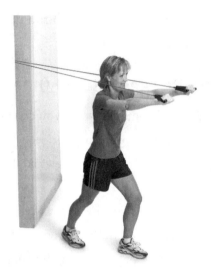

Here's how: First, secure your door anchor so that your tube is at about shoulder height. Grasp a tube handle in each hand and step away from the door, creating your desired resistance. Keeping your feet staggered, bring your hands up and out to the sides, creating 90-degree angles at your elbows. With your eyes open, head and neck neutral, and abdomen firm, slowly press the handles forward and squeeze with your chest muscles as you exhale. Pause, then return to the starting position as you inhale.

#2 BACK ROW
(BACK, SHOULDERS, BICEPS)

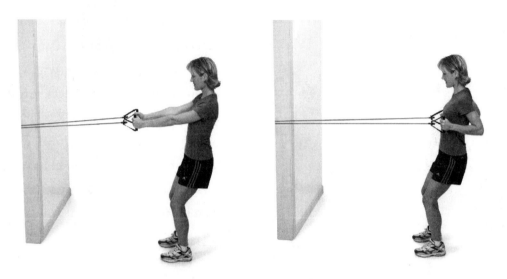

Here's how: First, secure your door anchor at waist height. Grasp a tube handle in each hand and step away from the door, creating your desired resistance. With your feet shoulder width apart, knees slightly bent, abdomen firm, and arms straight out, slowly pull the handles to your sides, squeezing your back muscles as you exhale. Pause, then return to the starting position as you inhale.

#3 TRICEPS PUSHDOWN
(TRICEPS)

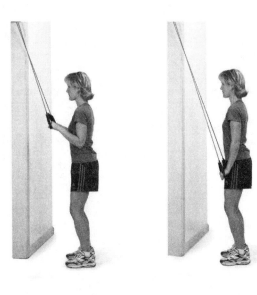

Here's how: First, secure your door anchor at the top of the door. Grasp a tube handle in each hand. With your feet shoulder width apart, knees soft, abdomen firm, and elbows at your sides, slowly push the handles down until your arms are straight as you exhale. Pause, then return to the starting position as you inhale.

#4 ABDOMINAL CRUNCH
(ABDOMINALS, LOWER BACK)

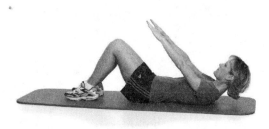

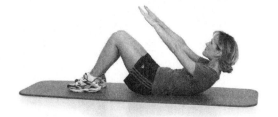

Here's how: Start by lying faceup, knees bent and feet shoulder width apart. With your eyes open and arms stretched out over your knees, slowly squeeze your abdominal muscles as you lift your head, neck, and shoulders no more than 6 inches off the floor as you exhale. Pause, then return to the starting position as you inhale.

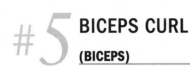

5 BICEPS CURL
(BICEPS)

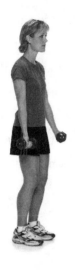

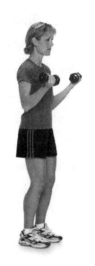

Here's how: Start by standing with your feet shoulder width apart, knees soft, and abdomen firm. Hold a pair of dumbbells that you can lift at your sides, with your palms facing forward. Slowly curl the dumbbells up toward your chest, keeping your elbows at your sides as you exhale. Pause at the midline of your chest, then return to the starting position as you inhale.

6 SHOULDER PRESS
(SHOULDERS, TRICEPS)

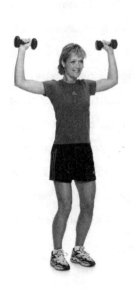

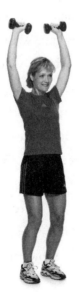

Here's how: Start by standing tall, feet shoulder width apart, knees soft, and abdomen firm. Hold a pair of dumbbells that you can lift over your head, then bring them up to the sides of your shoulders, elbows at 90 degrees. Slowly press the dumbbells over your head as you exhale. Pause, then return to the starting position as you inhale. If you want to add to the difficulty, try sitting on a stability ball while doing the exercise.

#7 BACK EXTENSION
(BACK, BUTTOCKS)

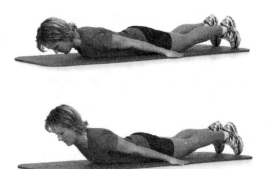

Here's how: Start by lying facedown on the floor with your arms at your sides, legs slightly apart, and eyes open. Slowly lift your head, neck, and shoulders as far as you can without hurting your back. Exhale, pause, and return to the starting position as you inhale. Don't strain your head, neck, or back.

#8 LEG SQUAT
(QUADRICEPS, HAMSTRINGS, HIPS)

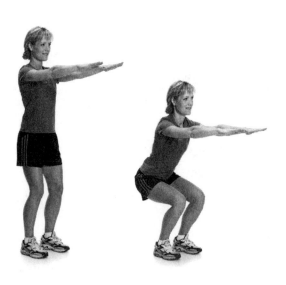

Here's how: Stand tall with your feet shoulder width apart, knees soft, abdomen firm, and arms straight out in front of you. With your eyes open, slowly start to bend your knees and sit down and back with your hips. Lower yourself until your hips are slightly higher than your knees as you inhale. Pause, then return to the starting position as you exhale. If you want to make this exercise a bit more challenging, hold a pair of dumbbells at your sides as you perform the same movement.

For Teenagers (Ages 13 to 17)

As your children enter their teen years, their bodies have already gone through considerable growth processes—forming the bones, joint sockets, muscles, ligaments, tendons, and height. Although genetics will ultimately determine fully grown musculoskeletal structures, it is safe to say that teenagers can begin to challenge their bodies now more than they could have before their 13th birthdays.

I recommend 3 days of strength-training exercises per week, doing one set of each exercise. Follow the number sequence from 1 to 8 to complete one go-round, or "circuit." Do 10 repetitions per exercise. If teens aren't strong enough to do 10 repetitions, they should do as many as they can. If your teenager wants more of a challenge, he or she can repeat the circuit of all eight exercises a second and even a third time, keeping the repetitions at 10.

Check your teenager's form at all times, and remember to consult your physician before your teen begins this or any other exercise program.

#1 CHEST PRESS
(CHEST, SHOULDERS, TRICEPS)

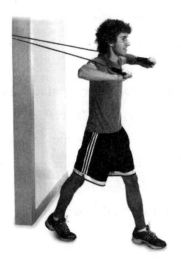 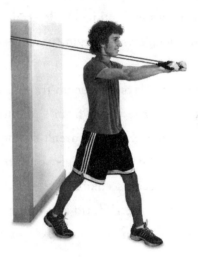

Here's how: First, secure your door anchor so that the tube is at about shoulder height. Grasp a handle in each hand and step away from the door, creating your desired resistance. Using a staggered foot stance, bring your hands up and out to the sides, creating 90-degree angles at your elbows. With your eyes open, head and neck neutral, and abdomen firm, slowly press the handles forward and squeeze with your chest muscles.

#2 BACK ROW
(BACK, SHOULDERS, BICEPS)

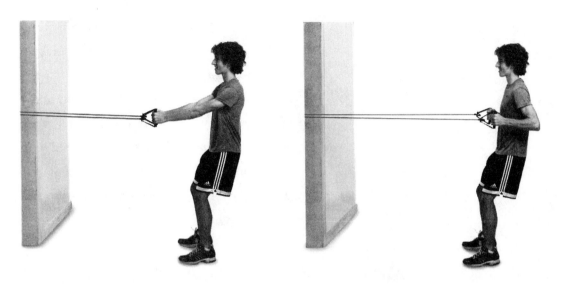

Here's how: First, secure your door anchor at waist height. Holding a tube, step away from the door, creating the desired resistance. With your feet shoulder width apart, knees bent, abdomen firm, and arms straight out, slowly pull the handles to your sides with your arms and squeeze your back muscles as you exhale. Pause, then return to the starting position as you inhale.

#3 TRICEPS PUSHDOWN
(TRICEPS)

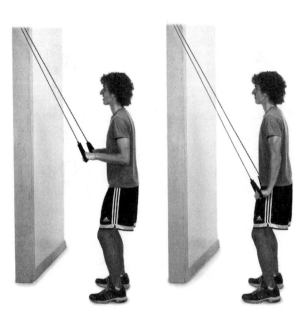

Here's how: First, secure your door anchor at the top of the door. Grasp a tube handle in each hand. With your feet shoulder width apart, knees soft, abdomen firm, and elbows at your sides, slowly push the handles down until your arms are straight as you exhale. Pause, then return to the starting position as you inhale.

#4 ABDOMINAL CRUNCH
(ABDOMINALS, LOWER BACK)

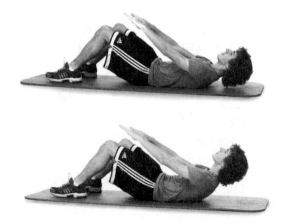

Here's how: Start by lying faceup, knees bent and feet shoulder width apart. With your eyes open and arms stretched out over your knees, slowly squeeze your abdominal muscles as you lift your head, neck, and shoulders no more than 6 inches off the floor as you exhale. Pause, then return to the starting position as you inhale.

#5 BICEPS CURL
(BICEPS)

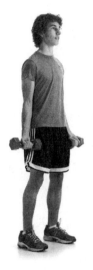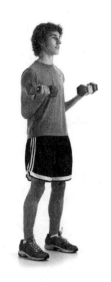

Here's how: Start by standing with your feet shoulder width apart, knees soft, and abdomen firm. Hold a pair of dumbbells that you can lift at your sides, with your palms facing forward. Slowly curl the dumbbells up toward your chest, keeping your elbows at your sides as you exhale. Pause at the midline of your chest, then return to the starting position as you inhale.

#6 SHOULDER PRESS
(SHOULDERS, TRICEPS)

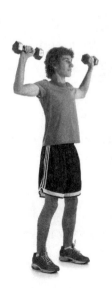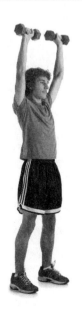

Here's how: Start by standing tall, feet shoulder width apart, knees soft, and abdomen firm. Hold a pair of dumbbells that you can lift over your head, then bring them up to the sides of your shoulders, with elbows at 90 degrees. Slowly press the dumbbells over your head as you exhale. Pause, then return to the starting position as you inhale. If you want to add to the difficulty, try sitting on a stability ball while doing the exercise.

#7 BACK EXTENSION
(BACK, BUTTOCKS)

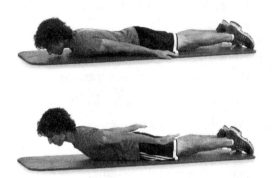

Here's how: Start by lying facedown on the floor with your arms at your sides, legs slightly apart, eyes open. Slowly lift your head, neck, and shoulders as far as you can without hurting your back. Exhale, pause, and return to the starting position as you inhale. Don't strain your head, neck, or back.

#8 LEG SQUAT
(QUADRICEPS, HAMSTRINGS, HIPS)

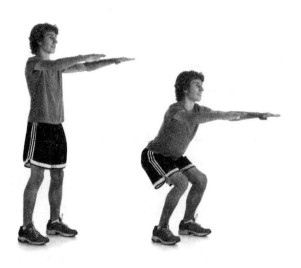

Here's how: Stand tall with your feet shoulder width apart, knees soft, abdomen firm, and arms straight out in front of you. With your eyes open, slowly start to bend your knees and sit down and back with your hips. Lower yourself until your hips are slightly higher than your knees as you inhale. Pause, then return to the starting position as you exhale. If you want to make this exercise a bit more challenging, hold a pair of dumbbells at your sides as you perform the same movement.

For Children (Age 12 and Younger)

For children, I recommend doing exercises that concentrate on pushing with their upper bodies, sitting and standing with their legs, using their arms and shoulders, and balancing on their feet. Along with their cardiovascular activities, boys and girls need just a little bit of resistance that will enable these foundation muscles to grow stronger. Kids 12 and under are too young to be lifting "weights." Misused and/or misguided weight lifting can possibly interfere with growth patterns or cause serious injury. Wait until your child is 13 or older to start using weights of any kind—and always provide proper instruction.

I recommend 2 days per week of strength-training exercises, doing one set of each exercise. Follow the number sequence to complete one go-round, or "circuit." Do 10 repetitions per exercise. Simply have your child follow the sequence of numbers from 1 to 7 to complete a full exercise session. Have your child complete all seven exercises at least once for a full workout. Kids should do anywhere from 1 to 10 repetitions, depending on their abilities. If your child is capable and wants more of a challenge, he can repeat the circuit of all seven exercises a second and even a third time, keeping the repetitions at 10. Check your child's form at all times and seek professional guidance if needed.

#1 PUSHUP
(CHEST, SHOULDERS, TRICEPS)

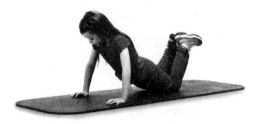

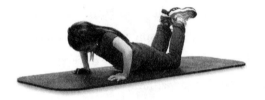

Here's how: Start by kneeling on the floor with your knees together. Lean forward and place your hands about shoulder width apart. With your feet in the air, slowly lower your body as you inhale. Stop when your elbows are at 90 degrees, pause, then push back up to the starting position as you exhale. Keep your upper body straight at all times.

#2 BACK EXTENSION
(BACK, BUTTOCKS)

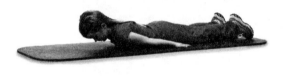

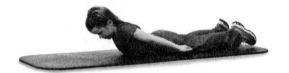

Here's how: Start by lying facedown on the floor with your arms at your sides, legs slightly apart, and eyes open. Slowly lift your head, neck, and shoulders as far as you can as you exhale, then return to the starting position as you inhale. Don't strain your head, neck, or back.

#3 BICEPS CURL
(BICEPS)

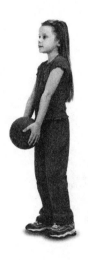 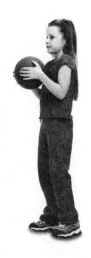

Here's how: Start by holding a light medicine ball or a rubber tube in your hands in front of your body, with your knees soft and feet shoulder width apart. Slowly curl the ball or tube up toward your chest, keeping your elbows at your sides as you exhale. Pause at the top, then return to the starting position as you inhale.

#4 OVERHEAD PRESS
(SHOULDERS, TRICEPS)

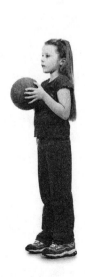 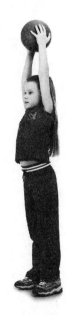

Here's how: Start by holding a medicine ball at chest height, with your knees soft and feet shoulder width apart. Slowly press the ball overhead as you exhale. Pause at the top, then slowly return to the starting position as you inhale.

#5 SIT/STAND CHAIR EXERCISE
(LEGS, HIPS)

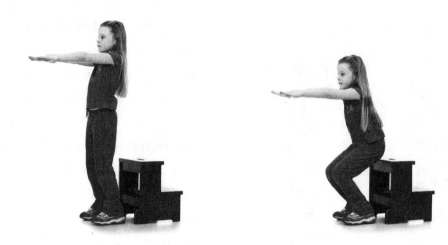

Here's how: Use a chair or step stool that you have to bend down to sit on. Stand approximately 6 inches in front of the chair. Slowly start to squat down toward the chair seat, keeping your chest up, back straight, and arms straight out in front of you as you inhale. Pause when the backs of your thighs or buttocks touch the chair, then return to the starting position as you exhale.

#6 ABDOMINAL CRUNCH
(ABDOMINALS, LOWER BACK)

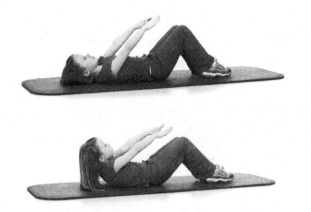

Here's how: Start by lying faceup on the floor, with your knees bent and feet flat and shoulder width apart. With your arms stretched out over your knees, slowly squeeze your stomach muscles and lift your head, neck, and shoulders off the floor as you exhale. Come up only about 6 inches, pause, and return to the starting position as you inhale.

#7 ONE-LEG BALANCE
(LEGS, HIPS—ANKLE/KNEE STABILIZERS)

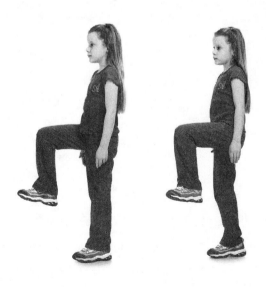

Here's how: Stand tall, with your feet 2 inches apart, shoulders back, chest up, and eyes open, facing straight ahead. Slowly lift one leg and bend the knee at 90 degrees. Keep the other knee soft, never locked. Pause, then return to the starting position. Repeat on the other side. Breathe normally throughout.

Remember to always exercise in a safe, open area. Use a reward system for effort and a job well done. Whether it's a raise in allowance, sleeping over at a friend's house, or a trip to an amusement park, it will reinforce your children's understanding of these healthy habits. They don't need a reward every day, but maybe on a weekly basis. A family meeting is the best time to provide these individual rewards and get the support of the entire family.

So in Week 2, you and your family members are adding just a handful of *strength-training exercises* to your *cardiovascular activities*. Here's a convenient grid to help you visualize how these quick and easy activities can fit into your weekly schedules. Every member of the family should take 1 day off each week from exercise routines.

In the chart below, I have shown day-by-day activities. It does not matter which days of the week you exercise, as long as you do the activities for the prescribed amount of time.

	CARDIO ACTIVITIES							STRENGTH TRAINING						
	M	T	W	TH	F	S	SU	M	T	W	TH	F	S	SU
Children 12 and younger	30 min	–	30 min	–	30 min	30 min	DAY OFF	–	10 min	–	10 min	–	–	DAY OFF
Teenagers 13–17	30 min	–	30 min	–	30 min	30 min	DAY OFF	–	10 min	–	10 min	–	10 min	DAY OFF
Adults 18 and older	30 min	30 min	–	30 min	30 min	–	DAY OFF	10 min	–	10 min	–	–	10 min	DAY OFF

Note: Random days were selected for example purposes.

FIT FAMILY ACTIVITY

Before we start with this week's activity, let's look back and see how last week went. Did your family participate in an active family get-together in Week 1? If you didn't, each journal will have an empty space, beckoning for an entry. The Fit Family Activity itself is very much of a support system, even if it isn't a big, organized activity. As long as there was a date, time, and place and most, if not all, family members attended, it should be recognized as an achievement. Remember, for each individual family member to be successful, you need the support of everyone in the family—no exceptions.

For Week 2, I want to suggest swimming for your family activity. Many of my clients and their families often have swimming get-togethers, and they really enjoy them. Besides the fact that swimming laps is the best calorie-burning cardiovascular activity we know of, swimming just makes the body feel great!

Swimming and aquatherapy are often practiced for healing injuries, easing lack of mobility for disabled individuals, and helping people exercise injury-free by taking pressure off the body's joints.

But swimming is also fun for the family. Plan a day at a public or private pool. In a private pool, you could play water polo, volleyball, or catch. In public pools, guidelines may be different, so have a lap contest, see who can swim underwater the longest, or learn different swimming strokes.

One of my clients likes to take her entire family to her health club for a swim, and she invites one or two other families along for the day. They pack a lunch and picnic baskets and swim for hours at a time while everyone has fun in the water. Of course, safety comes first, so always have good swimmers in the water, make sure lifeguards are on duty, and don't swim right after you eat. Wait 30 to 60 minutes.

If you live near the beach, and the season is right, there's nothing better than a day of swimming at the shore and playing in the sand. We all know how preoccupied children get with sand and how active we all become! You can play and do just about everything there.

Most communities have open swims at the Y, the local high school, the local park district, the community center, or a health club. If you don't have access to a pool, you could spend the day at an indoor gym, at a park, or in the backyard playing a family game of volleyball. Or choose another fitness activity from appendix B.

WEEK 2 FINAL THOUGHTS

Okay, that's it for Week 2. I leave the rest in your capable hands, Mom—or should I call you Coach? Week 1 was all about getting started. Week 2 is all about making corrections and staying on track. The cement of your foundation needs your help to harden, so be sure to highlight each family member's successes and ask them to "re-up" their commitment.

Put a successful second week together, and you and your family will be looking at a solid foundation and a finished basement. See you on the first floor of your new house next week!

WEEK 2 ACTION STEP SUMMARY

❑ Hold your Week 2 Fit Family Meeting.

❑ Review food diaries and exercise/activity journals.

❑ Make needed corrections in goals or strategies.

❑ Plan healthy menus for the week: focus on lunch.

❑ Add strength training to cardiovascular routines.

❑ Plan your your Fit Family Activity: family swim or volleyball.

❑ Schedule your Week 3 Fit Family Meeting.

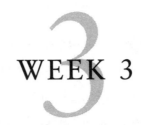

WEEK 3

Prevent Back Pain with a Strong Core

Two down—four to go! Are you excited? I am, that's for sure—because I know where you are in your journey. I know that a lifetime of good health, fitness, and managed weight control is just around the corner for you and your family.

JUST FOR YOU, MOM

Congratulations. You have 2 weeks under your belt—and speaking of your belt, it should be feeling looser now if you have been following my recommendations from Weeks 1 and 2. If you're not trimmer yet, don't panic. Those extra pounds didn't appear overnight, so they won't come off instantly either. However, this is a critical time for you to make sure you are following my recommendations for both food and exercise. Put one foot in front of the other, one block on top of the other, and your dreams will come true—I guarantee it.

You will lose weight this week, Mom, if you:

❏ Add one more strength-training circuit to your exercise session (increases calorie expenditure).

❏ Change your cardiovascular exercise to a different activity (gets results more quickly).

❏ Replace a candy bar snack with a piece of fresh fruit (saves up to 300 calories).

❏ Cut alcohol consumption by half (results in increased muscle hydration and weight loss).

Week 3 is a big one—there is a lot to cover, and you'll really need to have everyone's oars in the water. Let's go round up the troops for our Week 3 Fit Family Meeting.

WEEK 3 FIT FAMILY MEETING AGENDA

❏ Review food diaries and exercise/activity journals.

❏ Make corrections where needed.

❏ Discuss your meal planning and Week 3 Food Focus: dinner.

❏ Discuss and plan your Week 3 Fitness Focus: core exercises.

❏ Discuss and plan this week's Fit Family Activity: Get rolling.

❏ Schedule your Week 4 Fit Family Meeting.

WEEK 3 FIT FAMILY MEETING

Your Week 3 meeting discussion should start with you congratulating your family on the new healthy habits they're working to establish. Be sure that everyone stays committed to making healthier choices. If some family members are having a hard time keeping their motivation, encourage them by reminding them of their long-term goals.

REVIEW YOUR FOOD DIARIES

With 2 weeks now completed, you should be past the point of having to ask, "Are we filling out our food diaries and exercise/activity journals?" You should now be at a place where you are strategically using these tools to home in on your optimum healthy behaviors.

Hey, if we were all perfect, we wouldn't need these journals. But since we're not, we can all embrace the power of writing it down. Every slipup is important information, a guidepost to help us move in the right direction.

Close the Kitchen

Let's say that your food diary revealed that you were doing great all day—enjoying your light, wholesome meals; drinking plenty of water; getting a nice balance of lean protein and complex carbs. Then, at 9 P.M., your healthy day fell apart. You just couldn't stay away from the chocolate chip cookies or the pan of brownies. Since your food diary blew the whistle on this behavior, you can enlist some family support.

I recommend a task that young children can perform for the whole family: Post a sign on the refrigerator after dinner that says "Kitchen Closed." Although a child's task, the message is for everyone and must be followed by all. Many of us consume a disproportionate number of calories in the evening hours while we sit on the couch watching television. That is why the "Kitchen Closed" sign must be posted and taken seriously by all family members. Closing the kitchen after dinner may meet some resistance or cause some late-night sneaking at first, but stick with it. Once your habits change, those urges will diminish, and everyone's calorie count will too!

Check Water Intake

There are a couple more things I'd like you to review from last week's food diaries before we move on. First, look to see how everyone did with their water intake. Did they increase it and decrease the amount of sugary sodas? Look for any improvements, whether large or small. For example, if you were only drinking one or two glasses of water per day during the first week of the program, look to see if you're up to three or four glasses on an average day. If your kids don't like plain water, have they experimented with variations such as lemon water or cherry-flavored seltzer water?

Look at Portion Sizes

Another item to focus on is portion sizes. Check to see if everyone is being more careful about how much food is on their plates. Try portioning out food in the kitchen to avoid second helpings. Don't stand up to eat; sit down and enjoy your portioned meal or snack. Review your diaries to find portion-size issues and then come up with a solution for each person's situation. Refer back to Principle 2, "Manage Portion Sizes," for more advice.

Any Sticking Points?

Here at the start of Week 3, it's also a good time to ask everyone how they are doing in general. Check on all family members' energy levels, spirits, and frustrations. See if there are any sticking points. Altering food intake and activity habits can make people feel a little tired and sluggish. They may even see a change in their sleep patterns. Couple this with the rest of their hectic daily schedules, and you might have some very tired people. Be sure to inform your family that this is both typical and temporary.

At times, the human body will actually resist physiological change and become stubborn, holding on to both water weight and fat stores. But don't worry, this resistance is also temporary and will go away if you remain consistent with your food intake and exercise schedule. Slow, steady, moderate changes are the best method to use when it comes to healthy lifestyle habits, ensuring that they will become more effective and permanent.

Don't forget to use the family's support system to encourage any family member who is feeling challenged by the process. Again, lead by example and use other family members' successes, including your own, to help the members who need support.

WEEK 3 FOOD FOCUS: HEALTHY DINNERS

Dinner is the meal over which you have the most control. In many cases, the family is all together—at least a few times a week. You ought to use dinner as a central focus in your healthy eating strategy. It's usually the biggest meal of the day, so what your family does at dinner will have a major impact on the overall success of your week.

I'd like you to use dinners, especially in Week 3, to make sure that you're putting the basic food principles discussed earlier in the book into action. Ask yourself these questions: Are you managing your portion sizes? Are the kids drinking fewer sweetened drinks and more water? Are you incorporating lean protein and fiber into every meal? Dinner is also a good time to monitor how everyone in the family feels about healthier eating. You can get a pretty good idea just by observing how they are eating. Are they selecting food carefully? Eating at a relaxed pace? Being careful about how much food they are putting on their plates? Discuss what each family member has discovered about their eating habits over the past week, what they are most proud of, and what areas need work. Celebrate the successes and discuss solutions to any issues that continue.

Easy Meal Ideas

Does your family sit around the dinner table together and eat home-cooked meals? Do you go to a fast-food drive-thru? Do you just pick up the phone and order pizza? If you are like most families, it's a combination of all three. If your family is used to cooking most evenings, then the transition to the foods I've recommended probably hasn't been too difficult. However, if you have time-crunch issues, your family probably eats out a lot. Here are some quick, healthy, and family-friendly suggestions that are easy, affordable, and more nutritious than takeout.

- ❑ **Make-your-own-pizza night.** Use store-bought thin crust or whole wheat pitas. Add low-fat tomato sauce, a variety of veggies, and lean meat such as ground sirloin, low-fat sausage, or chicken. Add a small amount of reduced-fat mozzarella or freshly grated parmesan cheese. Bake at 400°F for 15 to 20 minutes.

- ❑ **Make-your-own-taco night.** Start with warm corn tortillas. Add canned refried beans (made without added fat), browned lean ground beef, chopped tomatoes, salsa, shredded romaine lettuce, sliced avocado, and shredded low-fat Cheddar cheese.

- ❑ **Sloppy Joe night.** Buy a large jar of Sloppy Joe sauce and add 1 pound of vegetarian meat crumbles or lean ground beef (for a family of four or five). Serve on toasted whole wheat buns with a fresh vegetable salad.

- ❑ **Pasta night.** Cook up whole wheat rotini (enough for 1 cup per person). Add your choice of low-fat Cheddar cheese or fresh parmesan (about 1 ounce per person) and stir in a variety of steamed vegetables, such as broccoli, asparagus, carrots, or cauliflower. Serve with baked chicken breasts (3 to 4 ounces per adult).

- ❑ **Homemade Asian-style stir-fry.** Buy precooked, frozen brown rice (⅔ cup per person) or prepare rice ahead of time. Serve it with stir-fried vegetables such as carrots, celery, soybeans, pea pods, onions, and sweet peppers. Add pork tenderloin or chicken (3 to 4 ounces per adult) with soy sauce.

- ❑ **Homemade chicken tenders.** Dip chicken breast strips (3 to 4 ounces per adult, 2 to 3 ounces per child) in beaten egg whites (2 per 8 ounces of meat) and coat with bread crumbs (⅓ cup per 8 ounces of meat). Bake at 375°F until crisp (about 20 to 25 minutes). Serve with fresh veggies and low-fat dip.

Follow these recipes to convert some of your family's favorite meals into "family fitness" meals. On the following pages, you'll find a week of Lean Mom, Fit Family meal ideas—breakfast, lunch, dinner, and healthy snacks.

WEEK 3 MENU PLAN

◆ = goal weight 160 pounds or lower

■ = goal weight over 160 pounds

● = kids age 12 and under

▼ MONDAY

Choose one option for each meal and snack.

BREAKFAST

High-fiber, high-protein cereal with milk

- ◆ ½ cup cereal, 3 tablespoons protein powder, 1 cup fat-free milk

- ■ 1 cup cereal, 3 tablespoons protein powder, 1 cup fat-free milk

- ● ½ to 1 cup cereal, ½ to 1 cup low-fat milk

Low-fat cheese melted on whole grain toast

- ◆ 2 ounces cheese, 2 slices toast

- ■ 2 ounces cheese, 2 slices toast, 1 cup fat-free milk

- ● 1 ounce cheese, ½ to 1 slice toast

Whole Wheat Pancakes (page 239), low-fat or vegetarian sausage

- ◆ 2 pancakes, 2 pieces sausage

- ■ 3 pancakes, 3 pieces sausage

- ● 1 or 2 pancakes, 1 or 2 pieces sausage

SNACK

Fruit Smoothie (page 263)

- ◆ ½ serving smoothie

- ■ 1 serving smoothie, 2 tablespoons protein powder

- ● ¼ serving smoothie

Celery with thinly spread peanut butter topped with raisins

- ◆ 1 rib celery, 1 teaspoon peanut butter, 1 tablespoon raisins

- ■ 1 rib celery, 1 teaspoon peanut butter, 1 tablespoon raisins, 1 ounce turkey

- ● ½ to 1 rib celery, ½ to 1 teaspoon peanut butter, ½ to 1 tablespoon raisins

Hard-cooked egg on whole grain toast

- ◆ 1 egg, 1 slice toast

- ■ 1 egg and 1 egg white, 1 slice toast

- ● ½ egg, ½ slice toast

LUNCH (EAT IN)

Minestrone soup, small whole grain roll, side salad with olive oil vinaigrette

- ◆ 1 cup soup, 1 roll, 1 cup salad with 1 teaspoon olive oil and balsamic vinegar

- ■ 1½ cups soup, 1 roll, 1 cup salad with 1 teaspoon olive oil and balsamic vinegar

- ● ¼ to ½ cup soup, ½ to 1 roll, ¼ to ½ cup salad with ½ to 1 teaspoon olive oil and balsamic vinegar

LUNCH (EAT OUT)

Boston Market rotisserie chicken, sesame broccoli, sweet corn

- ◆ 2 ounces chicken, 1 cup broccoli, ½ cup corn

- ■ 3 ounces chicken, 1 cup broccoli, 1 cup corn

- ● 1 to 2 ounces chicken, ¼ to ½ cup broccoli, ¼ cup corn

LUNCH (AT SCHOOL)

Zesty Tuna Salad (page 242), on whole grain roll, small apple, baby carrots

- ◆ ½ serving tuna salad, 1 roll, 1 apple, carrots

- ■ ½ serving tuna salad, 1 roll, 1 apple, carrots

- ● ¼ to ½ serving tuna salad, ¼ to ½ roll, ½ apple, carrots

SNACK

Low-fat cottage cheese with pineapple chunks and almonds

- ◆ ¼ cup cottage cheese, ½ cup pineapple, 8 almonds

- ■ ½ cup cottage cheese, 1 cup pineapple, 8 almonds

- ● 2 to 3 tablespoons cottage cheese, ¼ cup pineapple, 3 or 4 almonds

Trail mix made with Wheat Chex, peanuts or almonds, and raisins

- ◆ ¼ cup Wheat Chex, ½ tablespoon nuts, 1 tablespoon raisins

- ■ ½ cup Wheat Chex, 1 tablespoon nuts, 2 tablespoons raisins

- ● ¼ to ½ cup Wheat Chex, ½ tablespoon nuts, ½ to 1 tablespoon raisins

Low-fat vanilla yogurt, orange

- ◆ 1 cup yogurt, ½ orange

- ■ 1½ cups yogurt, 1 orange

- ● ½ to 1 cup yogurt, ¼ to ½ orange

DINNER

Lean roast pork tenderloin; Broccoli, Orange, and Watercress Salad (page 257); milk

- ◆ 3 ounces pork, 1 serving salad, 1 cup fat-free milk

- ■ 4 ounces pork, 1 serving salad, 1 cup fat-free milk

- 1 to 2 ounces pork, ¼ to ½ serving salad, ½ to 1 cup low-fat milk

Broiled tuna with fresh lemon, steamed broccoli, Wild Rice Casserole (page 254)

- ◆ 3 ounces tuna, broccoli, 1 serving casserole

- ■ 4 ounces tuna, broccoli, 1 serving casserole

- ● 1 to 2 ounces tuna, broccoli, ¼ to ½ serving casserole

Homemade Pita Pizzas (page 245), side salad with olive oil vinaigrette, milk

- ◆ 1 pizza, 1 cup salad with 1 teaspoon olive oil and balsamic vinegar, 1 cup fat-free milk

- ■ 2 pizzas, 1 cup salad with 1 teaspoon olive oil and balsamic vinegar, 1 cup fat-free milk

- ● ½ to 1 pizza, ¼ to ½ cup salad with ½ teaspoon olive oil and balsamic vinegar, ½ to 1 cup low-fat milk

▼ TUESDAY

Choose one option for each meal and snack.

BREAKFAST

Oatmeal with milk

- ◆ ½ cup oatmeal, 1 tablespoon protein powder, 1 cup fat-free milk

- ■ 1 cup oatmeal, 2 tablespoons protein powder, 1 cup fat-free milk

- ● ½ to 1 cup oatmeal, ½ to 1 cup low-fat milk

Low-fat vanilla yogurt with fresh fruit

- ◆ 1 cup yogurt, ½ piece fruit

- ■ 1½ cups yogurt, 1 piece fruit

- ● ½ to 1 cup yogurt, ¼ to ½ piece fruit

Shrimp and Veggie Omelet (page 240) with whole grain toast

- ◆ 1 serving omelet, 1 slice toast

- ■ 1 serving omelet, 1 slice toast

- ● ¼ to ½ serving omelet, ½ to 1 slice toast

SNACK

Low-fat vanilla yogurt mixed with frozen blueberries and sprinkled with 1 tablespoon sunflower seeds

- ◆ ½ cup yogurt, ½ cup blueberries, 1 tablespoon sunflower seeds

- ■ 1 cup yogurt, ½ cup blueberries, 1 tablespoon sunflower seeds

- ● ¼ to ½ cup yogurt, ¼ to ½ cup blueberries, 1 teaspoon sunflower seeds

One-half ham sandwich with tomato slices, sprinkled with lemon pepper

- ◆ 1 slice bread, 1 ounce ham, tomatoes

- ■ 1 slice bread, 2 ounces ham, tomatoes

- ● ½ slice bread, ½ ounce ham, tomatoes

Apple slices spread thinly with peanut butter

- ◆ 1 apple, 2 teaspoons peanut butter

- ■ 1 apple, 2 teaspoons peanut butter

- ● ¼ to ½ apple, 1 teaspoon peanut butter

LUNCH (EAT IN)

Chili made with lean ground beef, kidney beans, diced carrots, and green peppers; fresh orange sections

- ◆ 2 ounces beef, ½ cup beans, carrots, and green peppers, 1 orange

- ■ 3 ounces beef, 1 cup beans, carrots, and green peppers, 1 orange

- ● 1 to 2 ounces beef, ¼ to ½ cup beans, carrots, and green peppers, ¼ to ½ orange

LUNCH (EAT OUT)

Taco Bell beef burrito "Fresco style"

- ◆ ½ burrito

- ■ 1 burrito

- ● ¼ to ½ burrito

LUNCH (AT SCHOOL)

Turkey, lettuce, and tomato on whole wheat wrap, grape tomatoes, watermelon cubes

- ◆ 1 wrap, 2 ounces turkey, lettuce and tomato, grape tomatoes, 1 cup watermelon cubes

- ■ 2 wraps, 3 ounces turkey, lettuce and tomato, grape tomatoes, 1 cup watermelon cubes

- ● ½ to 1 wrap, 1 ounce turkey, lettuce and tomato, grape tomatoes, ¼ to ½ cup watermelon cubes

SNACK

Low-fat Cheddar cheese with whole grain crackers, apple

- ◆ 1 ounce cheese, 3 crackers, ½ apple

- ■ 1 ounce cheese, 6 crackers, ½ apple

- ● ½ ounce cheese, 2 or 3 crackers, ¼ apple

Fresh Homemade Salsa (page 260) with baked chips

- ◆ Salsa, 6 chips

- ■ Salsa, 12 chips

- ● Salsa, 6 chips

Low-fat vanilla yogurt with sliced fresh strawberries

- ◆ ½ cup yogurt, ½ cup strawberries

- ■ 1 cup yogurt, 1 cup strawberries

- ● ¼ to ½ cup yogurt, ¼ to ½ cup strawberries

DINNER

Roasted skinless chicken breast, Chickpea Salad with Red Onion and Tomato (page 256), milk

- ◆ 3 ounces chicken, 1 serving salad, 1 cup fat-free milk

- ■ 4 ounces chicken, 1½ servings salad, 1 cup fat-free milk

- ● 1 to 2 ounces chicken, ¼ to ½ serving salad, ½ to 1 cup low-fat milk

Grilled Salmon (page 245), baked sweet potato, steamed broccoli and cauliflower, milk

- ◆ 1 serving salmon, 1 small sweet potato with 1 teaspoon butter, broccoli and cauliflower, 1 cup fat-free milk

- ■ 1 serving salmon, 1 large sweet potato with 1 teaspoon butter, broccoli and cauliflower, 1 cup fat-free milk

- ● ½ serving salmon, ¼ to ½ small sweet potato with ½ teaspoon butter, broccoli and cauliflower, ½ to 1 cup low-fat milk

Lean beef hamburger, Baked French Fries (page 255), steamed carrots, milk

- ◆ 3-ounce hamburger, 1 serving fries, carrots, 1 cup fat-free milk

- ■ 4-ounce hamburger, 2 servings fries, carrots, 1 cup fat-free milk

- ● 1- to 2-ounce hamburger, ¼ to ½ serving fries, carrots, ½ to 1 cup low-fat milk

▼ WEDNESDAY

Choose one option for each meal and snack.

BREAKFAST

Whole grain frozen waffles, vegetarian or low-fat sausage

- ◆ 2 waffles, 2 pieces sausage

- ■ 3 waffles, 3 pieces sausage

- ● 1 to 1½ waffles, 1 piece sausage

Fruit Smoothie (page 263)

- ◆ ½ serving smoothie

- ■ 1 serving smoothie, 2 tablespoons protein powder

- ● ¼ serving smoothie

Breakfast Sandwich (page 237)

- ◆ 1 sandwich

- ■ 1 sandwich, 1 piece fruit

- ● ½ sandwich

SNACK

Spicy Bean Dip (page 261) with toasted small whole wheat pita and fresh veggies

- ◆ ¼ cup dip, veggies, ½ pita

- ■ ¼ cup dip, veggies, 1 pita

- ● 2 tablespoons dip, veggies, ½ pita

Low-fat cottage cheese with fresh cherries

- ◆ ¼ cup cottage cheese, 6 cherries

- ■ ½ cup cottage cheese, 12 cherries

- ● 2 tablespoons cottage cheese, 4 to 6 cherries

Apple Ladybug Treats (page 260)

- ◆ 1 serving treats, 1 ounce ham

- ■ 1 serving treats, 2 ounces ham

- ● 1 serving treats

LUNCH (EAT IN)

Veggie burger on whole grain bun with lettuce and tomato, baby carrots, grapes, milk

- ◆ 1 bun, 1 burger, lettuce and tomato, carrots, 15 grapes, 1 cup fat-free milk

- ■ 1 bun, 1 burger, lettuce and tomato, carrots, 15 grapes, 1 cup fat-free milk

- ● ½ bun, ¼ to ½ burger, lettuce and tomato, carrots, 6 to 10 grapes, ½ to 1 cup low-fat milk

LUNCH (EAT OUT)

Arby's roast beef wrap with light cheese and no sauce

- ◆ 1 wrap

- ■ 1 wrap, 1 cup fat-free milk

- ● ¼ to ½ wrap

LUNCH (AT SCHOOL)

Egg Salad (page 242) on whole grain bread, cucumber slices, red grapes

- ◆ 1 slice bread, 1 serving egg salad, cucumber slices, 15 grapes

- ■ 1 slice bread, 1 serving egg salad, cucumber slices, 15 grapes, 1 cup fat-free milk

- ● ½ to 1 slice bread, ½ serving egg salad, cucumber slices, 6 to 10 grapes

SNACK

Protein bar (14+ grams protein, 25 grams carbohydrates, less than 3 grams fat)

- ◆ ½ energy bar

- ■ 1 energy bar

- ● ¼ to ½ energy bar

Reduced-fat mozzarella sticks, fresh pear

- ◆ 1 cheese stick, 1 pear

- ■ 2 cheese sticks, 1 pear

- ● ½ cheese stick, ½ pear

Thinly spread peanut butter on whole grain toast, apple

- ◆ ½ teaspoon peanut butter, ½ slice toast, ½ apple, 1 ounce turkey

- ■ 1 teaspoon peanut butter, 1 slice toast, 1 apple, 1 ounce turkey

- ● ½ teaspoon peanut butter, ¼ to ½ slice toast, ¼ to ½ apple

DINNER

Grilled Salmon (page 245), steamed green beans, brown rice casserole with low-fat Cheddar cheese and steamed spinach, milk

- ◆ 1 serving salmon, green beans, ⅓ cup rice with 1 ounce cheese and spinach, 1 cup fat-free milk

- ■ 1 serving salmon, green beans, ⅔ cup rice with 1 ounce cheese and spinach, 1 cup fat-free milk

- ● ½ serving salmon, green beans, 2 to 4 tablespoons rice with ½ to 1 ounce cheese and spinach, ½ to 1 cup low-fat milk

Feta-Stuffed Chicken (page 247), side salad with olive oil vinaigrette

- ◆ ¾ serving chicken, 1 cup salad with 1 teaspoon olive oil and balsamic vinegar

- ■ 1 serving chicken, 1 cup salad with 1 teaspoon olive oil and balsamic vinegar

- ● ¼ to ½ serving chicken, ¼ to ½ cup salad with ½ to 1 teaspoon olive oil and balsamic vinegar

Black Bean Soup (page 248); sliced tomato, fresh mozzarella, and basil salad sprinkled with balsamic vinaigrette; milk

- ◆ 1 serving soup, tomatoes with ½ ounce cheese and basil, 1 cup fat-free milk

- ■ 1 serving soup, tomatoes with 1 ounce cheese and basil, 1 cup fat-free milk

- ● ¼ to ½ serving soup, tomatoes with ½ ounce cheese and basil, ½ to 1 cup low-fat milk

▼ THURSDAY

Choose one option for each meal and snack.

BREAKFAST

Breakfast Sandwich (page 237)

- ◆ 1 sandwich

- ■ 1 sandwich, 1 piece fruit

- ● ½ sandwich

Oatmeal with milk

- ◆ ½ cup oatmeal, 1 tablespoon protein powder, 1 cup fat-free milk

- ■ 1 cup oatmeal, 2 tablespoons protein powder, 1 cup fat-free milk

- ● ½ to 1 cup oatmeal, ½ to 1 cup low-fat milk

Low-fat vanilla yogurt with fresh fruit

- ◆ 1 cup yogurt, ½ piece fruit

- ■ 1½ cups yogurt, 1 piece fruit

- ● ½ to 1 cup yogurt, ¼ to ½ piece fruit

SNACK

Reduced-fat mozzarella sticks and raisins

- ◆ 1 cheese stick, 2 tablespoons raisins

- ■ 2 cheese sticks, 4 tablespoons raisins

- ● ½ to 1 cheese stick, 1 to 2 tablespoons raisins

Apple Ladybug Treats (page 260)

- ◆ 1 serving treats, 1 ounce ham

- ■ 1 serving treats, 2 ounces ham

- ● 1 serving treats

Veggie Dip (page 262) with fresh-cut vegetables

- ◆ 1 serving dip, veggies

- ■ 1 serving dip, veggies, 1 ounce turkey

- ● ½ to 1 serving dip, veggies

LUNCH (EAT IN)

Couscous with Portobello Mushrooms and Sun-Dried Tomatoes (page 241), grilled chicken

- ◆ 1 serving couscous, 2 ounces chicken

- ■ 1 serving couscous, 3 ounces chicken

- ● ¼ to ½ serving couscous, 1 to 2 ounces chicken

LUNCH (AT SCHOOL)

Roast beef sandwich on whole grain bread, side salad with olive oil vinaigrette, cantaloupe cubes.

- ◆ 1 slice bread, 2 ounces roast beef, 1 cup salad with 1 teaspoon olive oil and balsamic vinegar, 1 cup cantaloupe cubes

- ■ 2 slices bread, 3 ounces roast beef, 1 cup salad with 1 teaspoon olive oil and balsamic vinegar, 1 cup cantaloupe cubes

- ● 1 slice bread, 1 to 2 ounces roast beef, ½ cup salad with ½ teaspoon olive oil and balsamic vinegar, ¼ to ½ cup cantaloupe cubes

LUNCH (EAT OUT)

6" Subway sweet onion chicken teriyaki sandwich on wheat bread with 1 added fat (either cheese, oil, or mayo)

- ◆ 1 sandwich with 1 added fat

- ■ 1 sandwich with 1 added fat

- ● ½ sandwich with 1 added fat

SNACK

Edamame (soybeans)—buy fresh or frozen and boil. If precooked, heat in microwave.

- ◆ ½ cup edamame

- ■ 1 cup edamame

- ● ¼ cup edamame

Turkey sandwich with fresh tomato on whole grain bread

◆ 1 slice bread, 1 ounce turkey, tomato slices

■ 2 slices bread, 2 ounces turkey, tomato slices

● ¼ to ½ slice bread, ½ to 1 ounce turkey, tomato slices

Protein bar (14+ grams protein, 25 grams carbohydrates, less than 3 grams fat)

◆ ½ energy bar

■ 1 energy bar

● ¼ to ½ energy bar

DINNER

Chicken or tofu stir-fry with broccoli, water chestnuts, and carrots; brown rice; milk

◆ 3 ounces chicken or tofu with vegetables, ⅓ cup rice, 1 cup fat-free milk

■ 4 ounces chicken or tofu with vegetables, ⅔ cup rice, 1 cup fat-free milk

● 2 to 3 ounces chicken or tofu with vegetables, 2 to 4 tablespoons rice, ½ to 1 cup low-fat milk

Grilled lean steak, Roasted Vegetables (page 258), red potatoes

◆ 3 ounces steak, 1 serving vegetables, 1 cup potatoes

■ 4 ounces steak, 1 serving vegetables, 1½ cups potatoes

● 2 to 3 ounces steak, ½ to 1 serving vegetables, ½ to 1 cup potatoes

Soft tacos made with whole wheat tortillas, lean grilled steak or chicken, tomatoes and lettuce, and low-fat cheese; milk

◆ 2 tortillas, 3 ounces meat, tomatoes and lettuce, 1 ounce cheese, 1 cup fat-free milk

■ 3 tortillas, 4 ounces meat, tomatoes and lettuce, 1 ounce cheese, 1 cup fat-free milk

● 1 tortilla, 1 to 2 ounces meat, tomatoes and lettuce, ½ to 1 ounce cheese, ½ to 1 cup low-fat milk

▼FRIDAY

Choose one option for each meal and snack.

BREAKFAST

Breakfast Sandwich (page 237)

◆ 1 sandwich

■ 1 sandwich, 1 piece fruit

● ½ sandwich

Oatmeal with milk

◆ ½ cup oatmeal, 1 tablespoon protein powder, 1 cup fat-free milk

- 1 cup oatmeal, 2 tablespoons protein powder, 1 cup fat-free milk
- ½ to 1 cup oatmeal, ½ to 1 cup low-fat milk

Scrambled egg with whole grain toast

- 1 egg and 1 egg white, 2 slices toast
- 1 egg and 2 egg whites, 3 slices toast
- 1 egg, 1 slice toast

SNACK

Fun Fruit Kebabs (page 263) dipped in low-fat vanilla yogurt

- 1 kebab, ½ cup yogurt
- 1 kebab, ½ cup yogurt mixed with ¼ cup cottage cheese
- ½ to 1 kebab, ¼ to ½ cup yogurt

Apple slices with thinly spread peanut butter

- 1 apple, 1 teaspoon peanut butter
- 1 apple, 1 teaspoon peanut butter, 1 ounce turkey
- ¼ to ½ apple, ½ to 1 teaspoon peanut butter

Low-fat Jarlsberg cheese on whole grain toast, grapes

- 1 ounce cheese, ½ slice toast, 15 grapes
- 2 ounces cheese, 1 slice toast, 15 grapes
- ½ to 1 ounce cheese, ½ slice toast, 6 to 10 grapes

LUNCH (EAT IN)

Split pea soup made with ham, carrots, celery, and onions; small whole grain roll

- 1 cup soup (with 1 ounce ham), 1 roll
- 1½ cups soup (with 2 ounces ham), 1 roll
- ½ to ¾ cup soup (with ½ to 1 ounce ham), ½ roll

LUNCH (EAT OUT)

Chicken vegetable soup, small whole grain roll, side salad with olive oil vinaigrette

- 1 cup soup (with 2 ounces chicken), 1 roll, 1 cup salad with 1 teaspoon olive oil and balsamic vinegar
- 2 cups soup (with 3 ounces chicken), 1 roll, 1 cup salad with 1 teaspoon olive oil and balsamic vinegar
- ½ to ¾ cup soup (with 1 ounce chicken), ½ roll, ½ cup salad with ½ teaspoon olive oil and balsamic vinegar

LUNCH (AT SCHOOL)

Peanut butter and banana sandwich on whole grain bread (with natural peanut butter), grapes

- 1 slice bread, 1 teaspoon peanut butter, ¼ banana, 15 grapes
- 2 slices bread, 2 teaspoons peanut butter, ½ banana, 15 grapes
- ½ to 1 slice bread, ½ to 1 teaspoon peanut butter, ¼ banana, 6 to 10 grapes

SNACK

Turkey and low-fat cheese on whole grain crackers, dried apricots

- ◆ ½ ounce turkey, ½ ounce cheese, 3 crackers, 2 apricots

- ■ 1 ounce turkey, 1 ounce cheese, 6 crackers, 4 apricots

- ● ½ ounce turkey, ½ ounce cheese, 2 or 3 crackers, 1 apricot

Low-fat cottage cheese mixed with low-fat sour cream and sprinkled with cinnamon and brown sugar, with fresh fruit for dipping

- ◆ ¼ cup cottage cheese, 1 tablespoon sour cream, ½ cup fruit

- ■ ½ cup cottage cheese, 1 tablespoon sour cream, ½ cup fruit

- ● 2 to 3 tablespoons cottage cheese, ½ tablespoon sour cream, ¼ cup fruit

Fruit Smoothie (page 263)

- ◆ ½ serving smoothie

- ■ 1 serving smoothie, 2 tablespoons protein powder

- ● ¼ serving smoothie

DINNER

Grilled Beef Tenderloin (page 249), baked potato with low-fat sour cream, Roasted Asparagus (page 258), milk

- ◆ ½ serving beef, 1 small potato with 1 tablespoon sour cream, 1 serving asparagus, 1 cup fat-free milk

- ■ ½ serving beef, 1 large potato with 1 tablespoon sour cream, 1 serving asparagus, 1 cup fat-free milk

- ● ¼ serving beef, ½ small potato with ½ tablespoon sour cream, ½ serving asparagus, ½ to 1 cup low-fat milk

Roasted skinless chicken breast, red potatoes, steamed cabbage, milk

- ◆ 3 ounces chicken, ½ cup potatoes, ½ cup cabbage, 1 cup fat-free milk

- ■ 4 ounces chicken, 1 cup potatoes, ½ cup cabbage, 1 cup fat-free milk

- ● 1 to 2 ounces chicken, ¼ cup potatoes, ¼ cup cabbage, ½ to 1 cup low-fat milk

Quick and Spicy Fish Fillets (page 246), brown rice pilaf, Green Beans with Toasted Almonds (page 259), milk

- ◆ 1 serving fish, ⅓ cup pilaf, 1 serving green beans, 1 cup fat-free milk

- ■ 1 serving fish, ⅔ cup pilaf, 1 serving green beans, 1 cup fat-free milk

- ● ½ serving fish, 3 to 4 tablespoons pilaf, ½ serving green beans, ½ to 1 cup low-fat milk

Choose one option for each meal and snack.

BREAKFAST

Spinach and Feta Omelet (page 238)

◆ 1 serving omelet

■ 1 serving omelet

● ¼ to ½ serving omelet

French toast made with whole grain bread, vegetarian or low-fat sausage

◆ 2 slices French toast, 1 piece sausage

■ 3 slices French toast, 2 pieces sausage

● ½ to 1 slice French toast, 1 piece sausage

High-fiber, high-protein cereal with milk

◆ ½ cup cereal, 3 tablespoons protein powder, 1 cup fat-free milk

■ 1 cup cereal, 3 tablespoons protein powder, 1 cup fat-free milk

● ½ to 1 cup cereal, ½ to 1 cup low-fat milk

SNACK

One-half peanut butter and jelly sandwich with sliced strawberries (with natural peanut butter and all-fruit jam)

◆ ½ slice bread, ½ teaspoon peanut butter, ½ teaspoon jam, ¼ cup strawberries

■ 1 slice bread, 1 teaspoon peanut butter, 1 teaspoon jam, ¼ cup strawberries

● ½ slice bread, ½ teaspoon peanut butter, ½ teaspoon jam, 2 to 3 tablespoons strawberries

Hummus and fresh vegetables

◆ 4 tablespoons hummus, vegetables

■ 6 tablespoons hummus, vegetables

● 2 tablespoons hummus, vegetables

Low-fat vanilla yogurt with orange slices

◆ ½ cup yogurt, ½ orange

■ ½ cup yogurt mixed with ¼ cup cottage cheese, ½ orange

● ¼ to ½ cup yogurt, ¼ orange

LUNCH (EAT IN)

Wild Rice Apple Salad (page 255), grilled chicken breast

◆ ½ serving salad, 2 ounces chicken

■ 1 serving salad, 3 ounces chicken

● ¼ serving salad, 1 ounce chicken

Whole wheat pasta and tuna, steamed carrots, milk

◆ ½ cup pasta, 2 ounces tuna, carrots, 1 cup fat-free milk

■ 1 cup pasta, 3 ounces tuna, carrots, 1 cup fat-free milk

- ¼ cup pasta, 1 to 2 ounces tuna, carrots, ½ to 1 cup low-fat milk

LUNCH (EAT OUT)

Grilled chicken sandwich on whole grain bun, steamed vegetables

- ◆ 1 bun, 2 ounces chicken, vegetables

- ■ 1 bun, 3 ounces chicken, vegetables, 1 apple

- ● ½ bun, 1 to 2 ounces chicken, vegetables

SNACK

Veggie Dip (page 262) with fresh-cut vegetables

- ◆ 1 serving dip, vegetables

- ■ 2 servings dip, vegetables

- ● ½ serving dip, vegetables

Zesty Tuna Salad (page 242) on whole grain crackers, apple

- ◆ ¼ serving tuna salad, 3 crackers, ½ apple

- ■ ½ serving tuna salad, 6 crackers, ½ apple

- ● ¼ serving tuna salad, 2 or 3 crackers, ¼ apple

Fresh Homemade Salsa (page 260) with baked chips

- ◆ Salsa, 6 chips

- ■ Salsa, 12 chips

- ● Salsa, 4 to 6 chips

DINNER

Homemade Pita Pizzas (page 245), side salad with olive oil vinaigrette, milk

- ◆ 1 pizza, 1 cup salad with 1 teaspoon olive oil and balsamic vinegar, 1 cup fat-free milk

- ■ 2 pizzas, 1 cup salad with 1 teaspoon olive oil and balsamic vinegar, 1 cup fat-free milk

- ● ½ to 1 pizza, ¼ to ½ cup salad with ½ teaspoon olive oil and balsamic vinegar, ½ to 1 cup low-fat milk

Feta-Stuffed Chicken (page 247), side salad with olive oil vinaigrette

- ◆ 1 serving chicken, 1 cup salad with 1 teaspoon olive oil and balsamic vinegar

- ■ 1 serving chicken, 1 cup salad with 1 teaspoon olive oil and balsamic vinegar

- ● ¼ to ½ serving chicken, ¼ to ½ cup salad with ½ teaspoon olive oil and balsamic vinegar

Baked chicken strips, Baked French Fries (page 255), steamed cauliflower sprinkled with low-fat cheese

- ◆ 3 ounces chicken, 1 serving fries, cauliflower, 1 ounce cheese

- ■ 4 ounces chicken, 2 servings fries, cauliflower, 1 ounce cheese

- ● 1 to 2 ounces chicken, ¼ to ½ serving fries, cauliflower, ½ ounce cheese

Choose one option for each meal and snack.

BREAKFAST

Whole Wheat Pancakes (page 239), low-fat or vegetarian sausage

- ◆ 2 pancakes, 2 pieces sausage

- ■ 3 pancakes, 3 pieces sausage

- ● 1 or 2 pancakes, 1 or 2 pieces sausage

Ham and Vegetable Frittata (page 238) with whole grain toast

- ◆ 1 serving frittata, 1 slice toast

- ■ 1½ servings frittata, 1 slice toast

- ● ½ serving frittata, ½ slice toast

Oatmeal with milk

- ◆ ½ cup oatmeal, 1 tablespoon protein powder, 1 cup fat-free milk

- ■ 1 cup oatmeal, 2 tablespoons protein powder, 1 cup fat-free milk

- ● ½ to 1 cup oatmeal, ½ to 1 cup low-fat milk

SNACK

Low-fat cottage cheese with fresh pineapple

- ◆ ¼ cup cottage cheese, ½ cup pineapple

- ■ ½ cup cottage cheese, 1 cup pineapple

- ● 2 to 3 tablespoons cottage cheese, ¼ cup pineapple

Fun Fruit Kebabs (page 263) dipped in low-fat vanilla yogurt

- ◆ 1 kebab, ½ cup yogurt

- ■ 1 kebab, ½ cup yogurt mixed with ¼ cup cottage cheese

- ● ½ to 1 kebab, ¼ to ½ cup yogurt

Hard-cooked egg on whole grain toast

- ◆ 1 egg, 1 slice toast

- ■ 1 egg and 1 egg white, 1 slice toast

- ● ½ egg, ½ slice toast

LUNCH (EAT IN)

Creamy Cauliflower Soup (page 244), small whole grain roll, side salad with olive oil vinaigrette

- ◆ ¾ serving soup, 1 roll, 1 cup salad with 1 teaspoon olive oil and balsamic vinegar

- ■ 1 serving soup, 1 roll, 1 cup salad with 1 teaspoon olive oil and balsamic vinegar

- ● ¼ to ½ serving soup, 1 roll, ¼ to ½ cup salad with ½ teaspoon olive oil and balsamic vinegar

Tomato soup with whole grain crackers, baby carrots

- ◆ 1 cup soup (made with fat-free milk), 6 crackers, carrots

- ■ 1½ cups soup (made with fat-free milk), 8 crackers, carrots

- ½ cup soup (made with low-fat milk), 3 to 6 crackers, carrots

LUNCH (EAT OUT)

Chicken and vegetable stir-fry with brown rice

- ◆ 2 ounces chicken, vegetables, ⅔ cup rice

- ■ 3 ounces chicken, vegetables, 1 cup rice

- ● 1 to 2 ounces chicken, vegetables, 2 to 3 tablespoons rice

SNACK

Popcorn, turkey slices with fresh tomatoes sprinkled with lemon pepper

- ◆ 3 cups popcorn, 1 ounce turkey, tomatoes

- ■ 3 cups popcorn, 2 ounces turkey, tomatoes

- ● 1 cup popcorn, ½ ounce turkey, tomatoes

Celery with thinly spread peanut butter topped with raisins

- ◆ 1 rib celery, 1 teaspoon peanut butter, 1 tablespoon raisins

- ■ 1 rib celery, 1 teaspoon peanut butter, 1 tablespoon raisins, 1 ounce turkey

- ● ½ to 1 rib celery, ½ to 1 teaspoon peanut butter, ½ to 1 tablespoon raisins

Low-fat cottage cheese with fresh cherries

- ◆ ¼ cup cottage cheese, ½ cup cherries

- ■ ½ cup cottage cheese, ½ cup cherries

- ● 2 to 3 tablespoons cottage cheese, ¼ cup cherries

DINNER

Chicken Vegetable Stew (page 248), small whole grain roll, side salad with olive oil vinaigrette

- ◆ 1 serving stew, 1 roll, 1 cup salad with 1 teaspoon olive oil and balsamic vinegar

- ■ 1 serving stew, 1 roll, 1 cup salad with 1 teaspoon olive oil and balsamic vinegar

- ● ¼ to ½ serving stew, 1 roll, ¼ to ½ cup salad with ½ teaspoon olive oil and balsamic vinegar

Sloppy Joes (page 252) on whole grain bun, steamed broccoli, side salad with olive oil vinaigrette

- ◆ 1 bun, 1 serving Sloppy Joes, ½ to ¾ cup broccoli, 1 cup salad with 1 teaspoon olive oil and balsamic vinegar

- ■ 1 bun, 1 serving Sloppy Joes, ½ to ¾ cup broccoli, 1 cup salad with 1 teaspoon olive oil and balsamic vinegar

- ● ½ bun, ¼ to ½ serving Sloppy Joes, ¼ to ½ cup broccoli, ¼ to ½ cup salad with ½ teaspoon olive oil and balsamic vinegar

Stuffed Peppers (page 251), small whole grain roll, side salad with grilled chicken and olive oil vinaigrette

- ◆ 1 serving peppers, 1 roll, 1 cup salad with 3 ounces chicken and 1 teaspoon olive oil and balsamic vinegar

- ■ 1 serving peppers, 1 roll, 1 cup salad with 4 ounces chicken and 1 teaspoon olive oil and balsamic vinegar

- ● ¼ to ½ serving peppers, 1 roll, ¼ cup salad with 1 to 2 ounces chicken and 1 teaspoon olive oil and balsamic vinegar

FITNESS FOCUS

Before we begin a new Fitness Focus for Week 3, I want to make sure you have journaled your strength training and fitness activities for Week 2. If the journal is empty, or you were able to do only part of my recommendations, it's important to evaluate the scenario before moving on. Remember what your long-term goals are, then break them down to your short-term goals and refocus on your weekly strategies. This goes for individual activities as well as for your Fit Family Activity. Changing and developing new habits is challenging—we all know this. Keep your focus by writing down your exercise activities.

Week 3: Core Exercises

In Week 3, our Fitness Focus will be all about the core, or midsection. The core of the human body can be divided into three areas: the front of the core (abdominal muscles), the sides of the core (oblique muscles), and the back of the core (lumbar muscles). When these three areas collectively function properly, your entire body will perform better, whether for your daily activities or for sports.

The core is appropriately named: It is the center of the body and is functionally responsible for most of the body's movements. Many of us become caught up in wanting a six-pack and mistakenly overexercise the midsection by doing crunches and nothing

 SENA SAYS:
Take care of your core first, and then the sleek abdomen will follow.

else. This creates an imbalance that can ultimately lead to back problems. Getting a six-pack is more about food intake than it is about exercise. The abdominal muscles respond quickly to repetition, so they are easy to develop, but just because they are developed doesn't mean you can show them off. You have to have a low body fat percentage in your abdominal area. This happens when you exercise regularly and eat healthy and nutritious foods—which is what you're learning to do during this 6-week program.

Here's the best part: Each time you add a core exercise or two, you're replacing one of the previous core movements, so you'll get a more advanced exercise program without spending much more time. I haven't forgotten how busy you are! So let's keep moving—literally.

For Adults (18 and Older)

As you get older, your core becomes more and more important to your ability to live with a full range of motion and as little back pain as possible. At one time or another, we all have some sort of back pain, discomfort, or lack of mobility. We all know how debilitating it can be, making it difficult to work and live—not to mention perform sports or exercise routines. The older you get, the more you should pay attention to keeping your core healthy.

Within your strength-training circuit outlined in Week 2, #4 (Abdominal Crunch) and #7 (Back Extension) are both core movements. This week, let's substitute additional core movements in place of those exercises. Replace exercise #4 with both #4a and #4b in your routine, for variety.

#4a SIDE OBLIQUE CRUNCH

(OBLIQUES, LUMBAR)

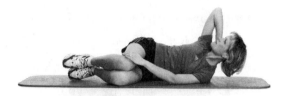

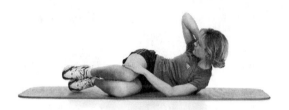

Here's how: Start by lying on your left side on the floor in the fetal position. Place your left hand on top of your right thigh for stability, and lightly place your right hand on the base of your neck. Remember to stay on your side. Looking up at your right elbow, slowly lift your head, neck, and shoulder toward your right hip. Exhale, pause, and return to the starting position as you inhale. Repeat on the other side. Be sure not to pull on your neck, and don't strain your head, neck, or back.

#4b REVERSE CRUNCH
(ABDOMINALS, OBLIQUES, LUMBAR)

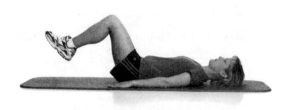

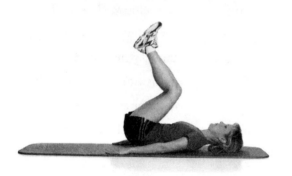

Here's how: Start by lying on the floor faceup, with your arms by your sides and your palms down. Raise your knees to a 90-degree angle over your hips. Slowly pull your belly button down to the floor and start to lower your legs, continuing until just before your lower back lifts off the floor. Pause as you inhale, then slowly raise your legs back up and over your abdomen, slightly tilting your hips up as you exhale and contract your abdominal muscles. Pause, then return to the starting position. Remember to keep your upper body stable and your eyes open, and pull your belly button down to the floor at all times.

When you come to #7 in your strength-training routine, replace it with these two core exercises, for variety.

#7a TUBE TWIST
(OBLIQUES, LUMBAR, BUTTOCKS)

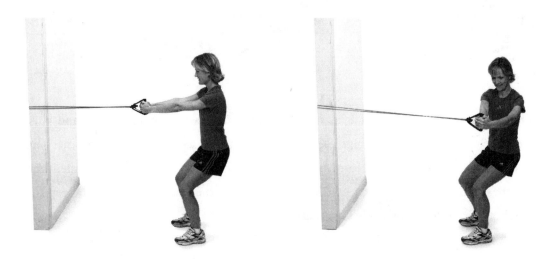

Here's how: First, secure your door anchor at waist height and attach a tube. Grasp both handles in your clasped hands and step back to create resistance. Next, stand facing the door with your feet shoulder width apart, knees soft, abdomen firm, eyes open, and head and neck neutral. Slowly turn your body to one side, then pause, exhale, and return to the starting position. Repeat to the other side. Remember to keep your arms straight and your feet pointed forward at all times while turning your midsection.

#7b LYING TORSO TWIST
(ABDOMINALS, OBLIQUES, LUMBAR)

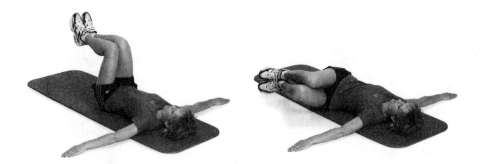

Here's how: Lie faceup on the floor with your hands out to the sides, palms down, and your knees bent at 90 degrees over your hips. Slowly lower your bent legs to the floor on either side as far as you can, stopping just before your legs touch the floor. Pause as you inhale, then return to the starting position as you exhale. Repeat to the other side. Remember to keep the opposite shoulder on the floor while lowering your legs.

For Teenagers (Ages 13 to 17)

During these years, your child's body will be able to take on more physical challenges as it grows stronger and becomes more agile and coordinated. Of course, motor skill abilities are different in every individual. This is a perfect time to teach and enhance skills such as agility, balance, and coordination. An effective method of teaching your kids to have better motor skills is to teach them to control their cores. If they can control their cores, they can control their movements.

Replace #4 (Abdominal Crunch) in the Week 2 strength-training routine with the following two movements, for variety.

#4a TRUNK TWIST WITH STICK
(ABDOMINALS, OBLIQUES, LUMBAR)

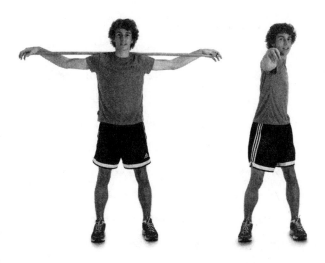

Here's how: Holding a broomstick or long dowel on your shoulders at the back of your neck, stand with your feet shoulder width apart, knees slightly bent, chest high, and arms draped lightly along the stick with palms forward. With your head and neck neutral and your eyes open, slowly rotate your body to one side, twisting your shoulders and torso while your head, hips, and legs stay straight ahead. Twist as far as you can without pain, then slowly return to the starting position. Repeat to the other side. Breathe normally and count 1 repetition each time you complete a twist to both sides. Do 10 repetitions.

#4b TOE TOUCH CRUNCH
(ABDOMINALS)

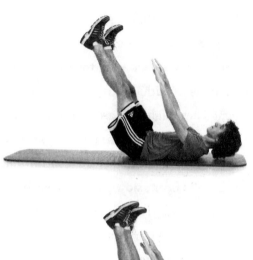

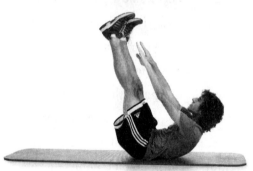

Here's how: Lying faceup in the same position as for the Abdominal Crunch, slowly raise your feet and hold them above your body. Pull your belly button down toward the floor as you contract your stomach muscles and lift your shoulders, trying to touch your toes with your outstretched arms. Exhale as you pause, then slowly return to the starting position as you inhale. Don't strain your head, neck, or back.

The same goes for #7 (Back Extension) in Week 2. This week, each time you come to #7, do the following two exercises, for variety.

#7a SUPERHERO
(BACK, BUTTOCKS, ABDOMINALS)

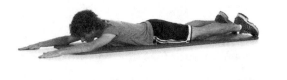

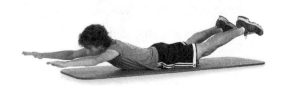

Here's how: Start by lying facedown with your arms on the floor by your head, with your palms down. Slowly lift your arms, shoulders, head, and legs as far as you can without straining. Exhale, pause, and slowly return to the starting position as you inhale. Keep your eyes open for equilibrium and your head and neck neutral.

#7b BENDING TOE TOUCH
(ABDOMINALS, LUMBAR, OBLIQUES, BUTTOCKS)

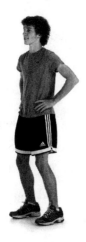 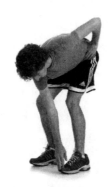

Here's how: Start by standing with your hands on your hips, feet shoulder width apart, knees soft, abdomen firm, head and neck neutral, and eyes open. Slowly bend over and touch your left toes with your right hand. Be sure to bend your knees and lower your buttocks as you reach for your toes (this will protect your back). Pause, then slowly return to the starting position. Repeat to other side. Breathe normally and keep your eyes open at all times.

These core exercises are very effective and more advanced than abdominal crunches and back extensions. Use caution and move slowly when performing these or any other exercises in this book. Proper instruction is always recommended, and have your doctor determine the health of your child's back before he or she performs these exercises.

For Children (Age 12 and Younger)

In the strength-training exercise circuit recommended for your children in Week 2, I have already included the right amount of core movements with #2, Back Extension, and #6, Abdominal Crunch. For this age group, those exercises are more than enough. Kids' cores will be directly and indirectly challenged and developed naturally through everyday activities such as running, jumping, skipping, and playing sports. So no extra exercises for these guys—just continue with strength training and sports.

Now, in Week 3, you and your family members have incorporated core exercises into your strength-training circuits, and it hasn't added any extra time to your busy schedule. Now that's what I call time management! Each time you and your family members do a strength-training circuit, you simply substitute the core movements, which will ultimately lead to a very healthy core and a trim waistline.

FIT FAMILY ACTIVITY

Mom, remember my three criteria for your family activity?

1. Perform together as a family.
2. Make it healthy.
3. Always have fun.

For Weeks 1 and 2, I recommended a soccer game and a swimming get-together. This week it's all about a bike ride. But it doesn't really matter what you do or in what order, just as long as you always meet the three criteria. The end result—a happier, healthier family whose members enjoy being together!

Biking is one of the world's most popular activities. It ranges from professional races to bike clubs to young kids with training wheels. Here in Week 3, I want to recommend a family bike ride. Of course, this will depend on everyone's schedule, so work with what you have. Think of a safe, close route. As I write these words, I'm looking out at a bright, sunny day and thinking of the many bike paths in the city of Chicago, where I live. I am always recommending that my clients take advantage of the great public parks in Chicago.

I'm sure you have lots of parks or bike paths to choose from that are fairly close to where you live, so think about where you and your family could ride for about 1 hour. Consider a path or an area that is not too crowded and has some slightly challenging terrain (gentle hills and curves) and a surface that's in good condition. A pretty setting always makes the ride more pleasant. Also, look for areas that have a place for you to rest and enjoy your healthy picnic lunch.

A bike ride like this can make for a couple of fun contests among family members. You could, of course, race each other—either for a long distance or in short sprints. You could also see who can balance the longest without moving! I love this one because it really challenges the body's core strength and stabilizing muscles.

If you pack a lunch, you could head to the park, zoo, botanical garden, or—my favorite—the beach for a picnic. Many beachfronts have great boardwalks for bike riding. Remember to pack a healthy meal with water bottles for all, cut veggies, lean meat or tuna sandwiches on whole grain bread, and fresh fruit for dessert. Stay safe by wearing helmets and making sure that all bikes have reflectors, mirrors, and sounding devices.

If it's too cold or rainy for a bike ride, get rolling inside. Find an indoor rink for an afternoon of roller skating. This is a fun activity with a great cardio benefit. It will also help with your balance and coordination, and it's always fun to compare the skills of kids and parents. Sorry, Mom, but kids usually have the edge here. (For more indoor ideas, see appendix B.)

WEEK 3 FINAL THOUGHTS

Think results! This is the week when you will start to feel and see the difference in your energy levels, your attitude, and potentially, your waistline. The key now is to form great nutrition and activity habits. Once you put them together, the end result will be a better, healthier you. The first floor of your house is looking good—keep hammering away.

WEEK 3 ACTION STEP SUMMARY

❏ Hold your Week 3 Fit Family Meeting.
❏ Review food diaries and exercise/activity journals.
❏ Make corrections with full family support.
❏ Plan your week of healthy meals, focusing on dinners together.
❏ Use dinnertime to observe family members' new eating habits.
❏ Integrate core exercises into your exercise routines.
❏ Plan your Fit Family Activity: family bike ride or indoor roller skating.
❏ Schedule your Week 4 Fit Family Meeting.

WEEK 4

Fight Disease with Five a Day

Congratulations—you've made it! You have reached the halfway point of my 6-week plan. You and your family members are all pulling the rope in the same direction. Nice going! You deserve a great deal of credit for making that happen.

JUST FOR YOU, MOM

For the past 3 weeks, you and I have had a little private dialogue between the two of us, where I've been sharing my best tricks of the trade. All of these healthy quick tips are designed to bring you results quickly and safely. And if you have been following my lead, you must be feeling and looking your best, or at least better than you have in a while.

I'm also proud of you if you've been *trying* your best but maybe have made some decisions that need to be reevaluated. If you haven't followed every recommendation perfectly, it's not about being "wrong" or "bad" or that you've "cheated." Get these negative thoughts out of your system now and forever. Lean Mom, Fit Family is a way of life. That means you'll be doing this for life without penalty or fault. When you have bad days, simply straighten things out and make better choices the next time.

Here at the start of Week 4 is a good time to encourage yourself and your family members who are in need. Remind yourself of your long-term goals, then your short-term goals, and then the strategies that will take you there. Refocus, that's all. We all need to do it.

You will lose weight this week, Mom, if you . . .

❑ Increase your strength-training repetitions by 5 to 15 per set (increases metabolic rate, which burns fat and sugar stores).

❑ Go up one more notch on the R.P.E. scale with your cardio exercise (turns up calorie burning).

❑ Cut intake of white flour products in half (refined carbohydrates can lead to sugar and starch cravings).

❑ Increase water intake by two or three glasses each day (flushes away toxins and decreases water weight).

You are leading the way and learning how to manage your own health and fitness as well your family's for the rest of your lives. I have some additional good news for you: The first 3 weeks, in my opinion, are more challenging than the next 3 weeks ahead of you.

Let me explain. During Weeks 1, 2, and 3, you and your family have been doing a lot of adjusting and schedule juggling to integrate new healthy habits into your lives, which is not easy. During Weeks 4, 5, and 6, you will continue to implement just a few new things each week. It will be easier because you have already formed new habits and have established your strategies and adjusted your schedules. In Weeks 4, 5, and 6, you will simply continue to put one foot in front of the other and keep it on cruise control. So let's go round up the crew for our Week 4 Fit Family Meeting and get them excited about their effort and progress.

WEEK 4 FIT FAMILY MEETING AGENDA

❑ Halfway summary—keep up the good work!
❑ Review food diaries and exercise/activity journals.
❑ Discuss progress—are we having fun?
❑ Discuss your meal planning and Week 4 Food Focus: fruit and veggies.
❑ Discuss and plan your Week 4 Fitness Focus: flexibility.

❏ Plan your Fit Family Activity: Take a hike!

❏ Schedule your Week 5 Fit Family Meeting.

WEEK 4 FIT FAMILY MEETING

Okay, let's start this meeting by encouraging everyone and letting them know how proud you are of them and their continued commitment and focus. You and the other family members have worked through some tough spots and worked out most of the kinks. It's time to measure your progress at the halfway point. Turn back to page 36 and have each family member take the Fit Family Quiz again. Then compare your scores to see how much your health has improved. Starting in Week 4, you should begin to see some real results!

Open up the meeting and allow your family members to discuss how they feel about the process. See if you can get everyone to talk about their successes and challenges. If the program hasn't taken hold with certain family members, you'll want to find the cause. I understand that we don't always embrace change, but try to put a positive light on anyone who may be falling behind. For example, if your daughter wants to lose weight and be more athletic so that she has a better chance of making the cheerleading squad, tell her to envision the fun that will come next season when she is on the sidelines cheering and hearing the applause of the crowd. Ask her why her progress has stalled and help her overcome her obstacles by reminding her that it really is all about showing up. If you can just get her to do that again, she will be on her way to success.

REVIEW YOUR FOOD DIARIES

Your food diaries should now be providing you and your family with a ton of insight into your individual food issues. There may be one or two of you who have nailed the meal plans and are feeling fantastic as a result—keep up the good work! Some of you may be halfway there and experiencing a taste of what it feels like to fuel your bodies on good, nutritious food. Regardless, you should all be very proud of yourselves for your commitment.

Here are the important points to look for from the past few weeks.

❑ Increasing water intake. Each family member should have added at least 1 to 2 glasses of water per day to be closer to your goal of 8 to 10 glasses per day.

❑ Carefully measuring and monitoring portion sizes and making behavioral changes that will move you away from overeating and toward a healthy view of food portions.

❑ Decreasing the amount of sugary drinks your family is consuming. It can sometimes take a while to get used to drinks that are not loaded with sugar, so be patient and stick with it.

❑ In your food diaries, look for signs of emotional eating patterns where you are using food as a coping mechanism, such as eating when you're under stress or feeling down. Work toward replacing overeating with more positive alternatives such as going for a walk, journaling your feelings, calling a friend, or deep breathing.

As you review your food diaries this week, check to see how many fruits and vegetables you are eating each day. If you're following my meal plan, you should already be at the recommendation of at least five servings of fruits and vegetables a day.

If you or anyone in your family is falling short, this week's food focus will help you reach optimum levels.

WEEK 4 FOOD FOCUS: FRUITS AND VEGETABLES

Our focus this week is on increasing the amount of fruits and vegetables in your meal plans to the ultimate goal of five or more total servings a day. As you may know, most Americans do not come close to this goal, and those who do often count ketchup and french fries as a serving (nice try!). However, fruits and vegetables are vitally important for their disease-fighting nutrients and their fiber content. In addition, I find that when people plan their meals and snacks around fruits and vegetables, other healthy choices tend to fall into place.

Planning your meals and snacks to include fruits and vegetables is a great way to help you reach your goals. Here is a variety of suggestions to get your children (and perhaps you and your spouse too!) to increase their intake of fruits and vegetables.

❑ Remember that it often takes many exposures before a child will try a new food. Be patient and continue to be a good role model in eating and offering vegetables, and eventually, the kids will come around.

❏ Serve lightly steamed vegetables with dips made with low-fat sour cream, cottage cheese, and veggie dip mix.

❏ Melt low-fat cheese on top of veggies to make them more appealing.

❏ Shred carrots and finely chop broccoli to stir into spaghetti sauce or pizza sauce.

❏ Add vegetables to soups, sandwiches, chili, and any other favorite recipes.

❏ Have your children pick out new fruits and vegetables at the grocery store.

❏ Go to one of the kid-friendly five-a-day Web sites (www.dole5aday.com, www.5aday.gov, www.5aday.com) and have your kids pick out a recipe. Taking ownership of the meal will make them more likely to eat it.

❏ Freeze fruits such as blueberries, grapes, and pineapple for a different kind of treat.

❏ Put cut-up fruit on skewers for fun-to-eat fruit kebabs. Serve with yogurt for dipping.

❏ Keep precut frozen vegetables in the freezer for a fast side dish.

WEEK 4 MENU PLAN

◆ = goal weight 160 pounds or lower

■ = goal weight over 160 pounds

● = kids age 12 and under

▼ MONDAY

Choose one option for each meal and snack.

BREAKFAST

Oatmeal with milk

◆ ½ cup oatmeal, 1 tablespoon protein powder, 1 cup fat-free milk

■ 1 cup oatmeal, 2 tablespoons protein powder, 1 cup fat-free milk

● ½ to 1 cup oatmeal, ½ to 1 cup low-fat milk

Whole grain frozen waffles, vegetarian or low-fat sausage

◆ 2 waffles, 2 pieces sausage

■ 3 waffles, 3 pieces sausage

● 1 to ½ waffles, 1 piece sausage

Breakfast Sandwich (page 237)

◆ 1 sandwich

■ 1 sandwich, 1 piece fruit

● ½ sandwich

SNACK

Veggie Dip (page 262) with fresh-cut vegetables

- ◆ 1 serving dip, veggies

- ■ 1 serving dip, veggies, 1 ounce turkey

- ● ½ to 1 serving dip, veggies

Trail mix made with Wheat Chex, raisins, and peanuts or almonds

- ◆ ¼ cup Wheat Chex, 1 tablespoon raisins, ½ tablespoon nuts

- ■ ½ cup Wheat Chex, 2 tablespoons raisins, 1 tablespoon nuts

- ● ¼ to ½ cup Wheat Chex, ½ to 1 tablespoon raisins, ½ tablespoon nuts

Reduced-fat mozzarella sticks with raisins

- ◆ 1 cheese stick, 2 tablespoons raisins

- ■ 1 cheese stick, 4 tablespoons raisins

- ● ½ to 1 cheese stick, 1 to 2 tablespoons raisins

LUNCH (EAT IN)

Black Bean Soup (page 248), side salad with olive oil vinaigrette

- ◆ 1 serving soup, 1 cup salad with 1 teaspoon olive oil and balsamic vinegar

- ■ 1½ servings soup, 1 cup salad with 1 teaspoon olive oil and balsamic vinegar

- ● ½ serving soup, ¼ cup salad with ½ teaspoon olive oil and balsamic vinegar

LUNCH (EAT OUT)

Wendy's Mandarin chicken salad (no noodles or almonds) with low-fat French dressing

- ◆ 1 salad, 1 tablespoon dressing

- ■ 1 salad, 1 tablespoon dressing

- ● ¼ to ½ salad, ½ tablespoon dressing

LUNCH (AT SCHOOL)

Turkey Apple Sandwich (page 243), baby carrots

- ◆ ½ sandwich, carrots

- ■ 1 sandwich, carrots

- ● ¼ sandwich, carrots

SNACK

Low-fat cottage cheese with fresh pineapple

- ◆ ¼ cup cottage cheese, ½ cup pineapple

- ■ ½ cup cottage cheese, 1 cup pineapple

- ● 2 to 3 tablespoons cottage cheese, ¼ cup pineapple

Low-fat cheese on whole grain crackers, apple slices

- ◆ 1 ounce cheese, 3 crackers, ½ apple

- ■ 1 ounce cheese, 6 crackers, ½ apple

- ● ½ ounce cheese, 2 or 3 crackers, ¼ apple

Spicy Bean Dip (page 261) with toasted small whole wheat pita and fresh veggies

- ◆ ¼ cup dip, veggies, ½ pita

- ◆ ¼ cup dip, veggies, 1 pita

- ● 2 tablespoons dip, veggies, ½ pita

DINNER

Cajun-Spiced Chicken (page 247), steamed fresh green beans, brown rice

- ◆ 1 serving chicken, green beans, ⅓ cup rice

- ■ 1 serving chicken, green beans, ⅔ cup rice

- ● ¼ to ½ serving chicken, green beans, 2 to 4 tablespoons rice

Grilled tuna steaks, whole wheat angel hair pasta with steamed asparagus and carrots, sprinkled with freshly grated Parmesan cheese

- ◆ 3 ounces tuna, ½ cup pasta with vegetables, 1 ounce cheese

- ■ 4 ounces tuna, 1 cup pasta with vegetables, 1 ounce cheese

- ● 1 to 2 ounces tuna, ¼ cup pasta with vegetables, ½ ounce cheese

Lean beef steak, succotash, side salad with olive oil vinaigrette

- ◆ 3 ounces steak, ½ cup succotash, 1 cup salad with 1 teaspoon olive oil and balsamic vinegar

- ■ 4 ounces steak, 1 cup succotash, 1 cup salad with 1 teaspoon olive oil and balsamic vinegar

- ● 1 to 2 ounces steak, ¼ cup succotash, ¼ to ½ cup salad with ½ teaspoon olive oil and balsamic vinegar

▼ TUESDAY

Choose one option for each meal and snack.

BREAKFAST

High-fiber, high-protein cereal with milk

- ◆ ½ cup cereal, 3 tablespoons protein powder, 1 cup fat-free milk

- ■ 1 cup cereal, 3 tablespoons protein powder, 1 cup fat-free milk

- ● ½ to 1 cup cereal, ½ to 1 cup low-fat milk

Low-fat vanilla yogurt with fresh fruit

- ◆ 1 cup yogurt, ½ piece fruit

- ■ 1½ cups yogurt, 1 piece fruit

- ● ½ to 1 cup yogurt, ¼ to ½ piece fruit

Spinach and Feta Omelet (page 238)

- ◆ 1 serving omelet

- ■ 1 serving omelet

- ● ¼ to ½ serving omelet

SNACK

Protein bar (14+ grams protein, 25 grams carbohydrates, less than 3 grams fat)

- ◆ ½ energy bar

- ■ 1 energy bar

- ● ¼ to ½ energy bar

Thinly spread peanut butter on whole grain toast, apple

- ◆ ½ teaspoon peanut butter, ½ slice toast, ½ apple

- ■ 1 teaspoon peanut butter, 1 slice toast, ½ apple

- ● ½ teaspoon peanut butter, ¼ to ½ slice toast, ¼ apple

Low-fat cottage cheese with fresh orange sections

- ◆ ¼ cup cottage cheese, 1 orange

- ■ ½ cup cottage cheese, 1 orange

- ● 2 to 3 tablespoons cottage cheese, ¼ to ½ orange

LUNCH (EAT IN)

Creamy Cauliflower Soup (page 244), side salad with olive oil vinaigrette

- ◆ ¾ serving soup, 1 cup salad with 1 teaspoon olive oil and balsamic vinegar

- ■ 1 serving soup, 1 cup salad with 1 teaspoon olive oil and balsamic vinegar

- ● ¼ to ½ serving soup, ¼ to ½ cup salad with ½ teaspoon olive oil and balsamic vinegar

LUNCH (EAT OUT)

McDonald's Chicken McGrill, side salad with Newman's Own low-fat balsamic vinaigrette dressing

- ◆ ½ sandwich, salad with 1 tablespoon dressing

- ■ 1 sandwich, salad with 1 tablespoon dressing

- ● ¼ to ½ sandwich, ½ salad with ½ tablespoon dressing

LUNCH (AT SCHOOL)

Egg Salad (page 242) sandwich on whole grain bread, grape tomatoes, red grapes

- ◆ 1 slice bread, 1 serving egg salad, tomatoes, 15 grapes

- ■ 2 slices bread, 1 serving egg salad, tomatoes, 15 grapes

- ● ½ to 1 slice bread, ¼ to ½ serving egg salad, tomatoes, 6 to 10 grapes

SNACK

Turkey sandwich with fresh tomato on whole grain bread

- ◆ 1 slice bread, 1 ounce turkey, tomatoes

- ■ 1 slice bread, 2 ounces turkey, tomatoes

- ● ½ slice bread, ½ ounce turkey, tomatoes

Edamame (soybeans)—buy fresh or frozen and boil. If precooked, heat in microwave.

- ◆ ½ cup edamame

- ■ 1 cup edamame

- ● ¼ cup edamame

Apple Ladybug Treats (page 260)

- ◆ 1 serving treats, 1 ounce ham

- ■ 1 serving treats, 2 ounces ham

- ● 1 serving treats

DINNER

Chicken or tofu stir-fry with broccoli, carrots, and water chestnuts; brown rice; milk

- ◆ 3 ounces chicken or tofu, vegetables, ⅓ cup rice, 1 cup fat-free milk

- ■ 4 ounces chicken or tofu, vegetables, ⅔ cup rice, 1 cup fat-free milk

- ● 1 to 2 ounces chicken or tofu, vegetables, 2 to 3 tablespoons rice, ½ to 1 cup low-fat milk

Asian Steak (page 253), brown rice

- ◆ 1 serving steak, ⅓ cup rice

- ■ 1 serving steak, ⅔ cup rice

- ● ¼ to ½ serving steak, 2 to 3 tablespoons rice

Soft tacos made with whole wheat tortillas, lean grilled steak or chicken, tomatoes and lettuce, and low-fat cheese; milk

- ◆ 2 tortillas, 3 ounces meat, tomatoes and lettuce, 1 ounce cheese, 1 cup fat-free milk

- ■ 3 tortillas, 4 ounces meat, tomatoes and lettuce, 1 ounce cheese, 1 cup fat-free milk

- ● 1 tortilla, 1 to 2 ounces meat, tomatoes and lettuce, ½ to 1 ounce cheese, ½ to 1 cup low-fat milk

▼ WEDNESDAY

Choose one option for each meal and snack.

BREAKFAST

Low-fat vanilla yogurt with orange slices

- ◆ 1 cup yogurt, ½ orange

- ■ 1½ cups yogurt, 1 orange

- ● ½ to 1 cup yogurt, ¼ to ½ orange

French toast made with whole grain bread, low-fat or vegetarian sausage

- ◆ 2 slices French toast, 1 piece sausage

- ■ 3 slices French toast, 2 pieces sausage

- ● ½ to 1 slice French toast, 1 piece sausage

Shrimp and Veggie Omelet (page 240) with whole grain toast

- ◆ 1 serving omelet, 1 slice toast

- ■ 1 serving omelet, 1 slice toast

- ● ¼ to ½ serving omelet, ½ to 1 slice toast

SNACK

Fruit Smoothie (page 263)

- ◆ ½ serving smoothie

- ■ 1 serving smoothie, 2 tablespoons protein powder

- ● ¼ serving smoothie

Low-fat cottage cheese with fresh cherries

- ◆ ¼ cup cottage cheese, ½ cup cherries

- ■ ½ cup cottage cheese, ½ cup cherries

- ● 2 to 3 tablespoons cottage cheese, ¼ cup cherries

Celery with thinly spread peanut butter topped with raisins

- ◆ 1 rib celery, 1 teaspoon peanut butter, 1 tablespoon raisins

- ■ 1 rib celery, 1 teaspoon peanut butter, 1 tablespoon raisins, 1 ounce turkey

- ● ½ to 1 rib celery, ½ to 1 teaspoon peanut butter, ½ to 1 tablespoon raisins

LUNCH (EAT IN)

Chicken Vegetable Stew (page 248), small whole grain roll, salad with olive oil vinaigrette

- ◆ 1 serving stew, 1 roll, 1 cup salad with 1 teaspoon olive oil and balsamic vinegar

- ■ 1 serving stew, 1 roll, 1 cup salad with 1 teaspoon olive oil and balsamic vinegar

- ● ¼ to ½ serving stew, 1 roll, ¼ to ½ cup salad with ½ teaspoon olive oil and balsamic vinegar

LUNCH (EAT OUT)

Arby's turkey wrap with no sauce, side salad with low-fat dressing

- ◆ ½ wrap, salad with 1 tablespoon dressing

- ■ 1 wrap, salad with 1 tablespoon dressing

- ● ¼ to ½ wrap, ¼ to ½ salad with ½ tablespoon dressing

LUNCH (AT SCHOOL)

Turkey wrap with lettuce, tomato, and cucumber slices in whole wheat tortilla (can use low-fat ranch dressing on the side); orange slices

- ◆ 1 tortilla, 2 ounces turkey, lettuce, tomato, and cucumber slices, 2 tablespoons dressing, ½ orange

- ■ 2 tortillas, with 3 ounces turkey, lettuce, tomato, and cucumber slices, 2 tablespoons dressing, ½ orange

- ● ½ tortilla, 1 to 2 ounces turkey, lettuce, tomato, and cucumber slices, 1 tablespoon dressing, ¼ to ½ orange

SNACK

Fun Fruit Kebabs (page 263) dipped in low-fat vanilla yogurt

- ◆ 1 kebab, ½ cup yogurt

- ■ 1 kebab, ½ cup yogurt mixed with ¼ cup cottage cheese

- ● ½ to 1 kebab, ¼ to ½ cup yogurt

Turkey and low-fat cheese slices on whole grain crackers, dried apricots

- ◆ ½ ounce turkey, ½ ounce cheese, 3 crackers, 2 apricots

- ■ 1 ounce turkey, 1 ounce cheese, 6 crackers, 4 apricots

- ½ ounce turkey, ½ ounce cheese, 2 or 3 crackers, 1 apricot

Hummus and fresh vegetables

- ◆ 4 tablespoons hummus, vegetables

- ■ 6 tablespoons hummus, vegetables

- ● 2 tablespoons hummus, vegetables

DINNER

Lean roast pork tenderloin with apple slices, steamed broccoli and cauliflower

- ◆ 3 ounces pork, 1 apple, broccoli and cauliflower

- ■ 4 ounces pork, 1 apple, broccoli and cauliflower, 1 small whole grain roll

- ● 1 to 2 ounces pork, ¼ to ½ apple, broccoli and cauliflower

Baked Fish with Vegetables (page 250), whole wheat rotini with freshly grated Parmesan cheese

- ◆ 1 serving fish with vegetables, ½ cup rotini, 1 ounce cheese

- ■ 1 serving fish with vegetables, 1 cup rotini, 1 ounce cheese

- ● ½ serving fish with vegetables, ¼ cup rotini, ½ to 1 ounce cheese

Homemade Pita Pizzas (page 245), side salad with olive oil vinaigrette, milk

- ◆ 1 pizza, 1 cup salad with 1 teaspoon olive oil and balsamic vinegar, 1 cup fat-free milk

- ■ 2 pizzas, 1 cup salad with 1 teaspoon olive oil and balsamic vinegar, 1 cup fat-free milk

- ● ½ to 1 pizza, ¼ to ½ cup salad with ½ teaspoon olive oil and balsamic vinegar, ½ to 1 cup low-fat milk

▼ THURSDAY

Choose one option for each meal and snack.

BREAKFAST

Oatmeal with milk

- ◆ ½ cup oatmeal, 1 tablespoon protein powder, 1 cup fat-free milk

- ■ 1 cup oatmeal, 2 tablespoons protein powder, 1 cup fat-free milk

- ● ½ to 1 cup oatmeal, ½ to 1 cup low-fat milk

Whole grain frozen waffles, vegetarian or low-fat sausage

- ◆ 2 waffles, 2 pieces sausage

- ■ 3 waffles, 3 pieces sausage

- ● 1 to 1½ waffles, 1 piece sausage

Low-fat cheese melted on whole grain toast

- ◆ 2 ounces cheese, 2 slices toast

■ 2 ounces cheese, 2 slices toast, 1 cup fat-free milk

● 1 ounce cheese, ½ to 1 slice toast

SNACK

Trail mix made with Wheat Chex, raisins, and peanuts or almonds

◆ ¼ cup Wheat Chex, 1 tablespoon raisins, ½ tablespoon nuts

■ ½ cup Wheat Chex, 2 tablespoons raisins, 1 tablespoon nuts

● ¼ to ½ cup Wheat Chex, ½ to 1 tablespoon raisins, ½ tablespoon nuts

Reduced-fat mozzarella sticks with raisins

◆ 1 cheese stick, 2 tablespoons raisins

■ 2 cheese sticks, 4 tablespoons raisins

● ½ to 1 cheese stick, 1 to 2 tablespoons raisins

Low-fat cottage cheese with fresh pineapple

◆ ¼ cup cottage cheese, ½ cup pineapple

■ ½ cup cottage cheese, 1 cup pineapple

● 2 to 3 tablespoons cottage cheese, ¼ cup pineapple

LUNCH (EAT IN)

Wild Rice Apple Salad (page 255), grilled chicken breast

◆ ½ serving salad, 2 ounces chicken

■ 1 serving salad, 3 ounces chicken

● ¼ serving salad, 1 ounce chicken

LUNCH (EAT OUT)

Taco Bell steak burrito supreme "Fresco style"

◆ 1 burrito

■ 1 burrito

● ¼ to ½ burrito

LUNCH (AT SCHOOL)

Low-fat cheese, turkey, and tomato sandwich on whole wheat pita with Dijon mustard; apple slices; baby carrots

◆ 1 pita, 1 ounce cheese, 1 ounce turkey, tomato, 1 apple, carrots

■ 1 to 1½ pitas, 1 ounce cheese, 2 ounces turkey, tomato, 1 apple, carrots

● ½ pita, ½ ounce cheese, ½ to 1 ounce turkey, tomato, ¼ to ½ apple, carrots

SNACK

Veggie Dip (page 262) with fresh-cut vegetables

◆ 1 serving dip, vegetables

■ 2 servings dip, vegetables

● ½ serving dip, vegetables

Low-fat cottage cheese mixed with low-fat sour cream and sprinkled with cinnamon and brown sugar, with fresh fruit for dipping

◆ ¼ cup cottage cheese, 1 tablespoon sour cream, ½ cup fruit

- ½ cup cottage cheese, 1 tablespoon sour cream, ½ cup fruit

- 2 to 3 tablespoons cottage cheese, ½ tablespoon sour cream, ¼ cup fruit

Protein bar (14+ grams protein, 25 grams carbohydrates, less than 3 grams fat)

- ♦ ½ energy bar

- ■ 1 energy bar

- ● ¼ to ½ energy bar

DINNER

Veggie burger on whole grain bun, Baked French Fries made with sweet potatoes (page 255), broccoli sprinkled with low-fat cheese

- ♦ 1 bun, 1 burger, 1 serving fries, broccoli with 1 ounce cheese

- ■ 1 bun, 1 burger, 2 servings fries, broccoli with 1 ounce cheese

- ¼ to ½ bun, ¼ to ½ burger, ½ serving fries, broccoli with ½ to 1 ounce cheese

Grilled Salmon (page 245), Sweet Carrot Salad (page 257), Wild Rice Casserole (page 254)

- ♦ 1 serving salmon, 1 serving salad, 1 serving casserole

- ■ 1 serving salmon, 1½ servings salad, 1½ servings casserole

- ● ½ serving salmon, ¼ to ½ serving salad, ¼ to ½ serving casserole

Cabbage Roll-Ups (page 249), side salad with olive oil vinaigrette

- ♦ 1 serving roll-ups, 1 cup salad with 1 teaspoon olive oil and balsamic vinegar

- ■ 1½ servings roll-ups, 1 cup salad with 1 teaspoon olive oil and balsamic vinegar

- ● ¼ to ½ serving roll-ups, ¼ to ½ cup salad with ½ teaspoon olive oil and balsamic vinegar

▼ FRIDAY

Choose one option for each meal and snack.

BREAKFAST

High-fiber, high-protein cereal with milk

- ♦ ½ cup cereal, 3 tablespoons protein powder, 1 cup fat-free milk

- ■ 1 cup cereal, 3 tablespoons protein powder, 1 cup fat-free milk

- ● ½ to 1 cup cereal, ½ to 1 cup low-fat milk

Low-fat vanilla yogurt with sliced strawberries

- ♦ 1 cup yogurt, ½ cup strawberries

- ■ 1½ cups yogurt, 1 cup strawberries

- ● ½ to 1 cup yogurt, ¼ cup strawberries

Scrambled egg with whole grain toast

- ♦ 1 egg and 1 egg white, 2 slices toast

- 1 egg and 2 egg whites, 3 slices toast

- 1 egg, 1 slice toast

SNACK

Spiced Pumpkin Seeds (page 262) and raisins

- ♦ ¼ cup pumpkin seeds, 1 tablespoon raisins

- ▪ ¼ cup pumpkin seeds, 3 tablespoons raisins

- ● 2 to 3 tablespoons pumpkin seeds, 1 to 2 tablespoons raisins

Apple slices spread thinly with peanut butter

- ♦ 1 apple, 2 teaspoons peanut butter

- ▪ 1 apple, 2 teaspoons peanut butter

- ● ¼ to ½ apple, 1 teaspoon peanut butter

Hummus with fresh vegetables

- ♦ 4 tablespoons hummus, vegetables

- ▪ 6 tablespoons hummus, vegetables

- ● 2 tablespoons hummus, vegetables

LUNCH (EAT IN)

Chickpea Salad with Red Onion and Tomato (page 256) with tuna

- ♦ 1 serving salad, 2 ounces tuna

- ▪ 1½ servings salad, 3 ounces tuna

- ● ¼ to ½ serving salad, 1 to 2 ounces tuna

LUNCH (EAT OUT)

Subway ham sandwich wrap

- ♦ 1 wrap

- ▪ 1 wrap

- ● ¼ to ½ wrap

LUNCH (AT SCHOOL)

Vegetable Sandwich (page 243), milk

- ♦ 1 sandwich, 1 cup fat-free milk

- ▪ 1 sandwich, 1 cup fat-free milk

- ● ¼ to ½ sandwich, ½ to 1 cup low-fat milk

SNACK

Fresh Homemade Salsa (page 260) with baked chips

- ♦ Salsa, 6 chips

- ▪ Salsa, 12 chips

- ● Salsa, 6 chips

Edamame (soybeans)—buy fresh or frozen and boil. If precooked, heat in microwave.

- ♦ ½ cup edamame

- ▪ 1 cup edamame

- ● ¼ cup edamame

Zesty Tuna Salad (page 242) on whole grain crackers, apple

- ♦ ¼ serving tuna, 3 crackers, ½ apple

- ▪ ½ serving tuna, 6 crackers, ½ apple

- ● ¼ serving tuna, 2 or 3 crackers, ¼ apple

DINNER

Lean beef hamburger on whole grain bun, Coleslaw Salad (page 259), milk

- ◆ 1 bun, 3-ounce hamburger, 1 serving coleslaw, 1 cup fat-free milk

- ■ 1 bun, 4-ounce hamburger, 1½ servings coleslaw, 1 cup fat-free milk

- ● ½ bun, 1- to 2-ounce hamburger, ½ serving coleslaw, ½ to 1 cup low-fat milk

Homemade Pita Pizzas (page 245), side salad with olive oil vinaigrette, milk

- ◆ 1 pizza, 1 cup salad with 1 teaspoon olive oil and balsamic vinegar, 1 cup fat-free milk

- ■ 2 pizzas, 1 cup salad with 1 teaspoon olive oil and balsamic vinegar, 1 cup fat-free milk

- ● ½ to 1 pizza, ¼ to ½ cup salad with ½ teaspoon olive oil and balsamic vinegar, 1 cup low-fat milk

Cajun-Spiced Chicken (page 247), brown rice, steamed green beans, milk

- ◆ 1 serving chicken, ⅓ cup rice, green beans, 1 cup fat-free milk

- ■ 1 serving chicken, ⅔ cup rice, green beans, 1 cup fat-free milk

- ● ¼ to ½ serving chicken, ⅓ cup rice, green beans, 1 cup low-fat milk

▼ SATURDAY

Choose one option for each meal and snack.

BREAKFAST

Whole Wheat Pancakes (page 239) with low-fat or vegetarian sausage

- ◆ 2 pancakes, 2 pieces sausage

- ■ 3 pancakes, 3 pieces sausage

- ● 1 or 2 pancakes, 1 or 2 pieces sausage

Ham and Vegetable Frittata (page 238) with whole grain toast

- ◆ 1 serving frittata, 1 slice toast

- ■ 1½ servings frittata, 1 slice toast

- ● ½ serving frittata, ½ slice toast

Oatmeal with milk

- ◆ ½ cup oatmeal, 1 tablespoon protein powder, 1 cup fat-free milk

- ■ 1 cup oatmeal, 2 tablespoons protein powder, 1 cup fat-free milk

- ● ½ to 1 cup oatmeal, ½ to 1 cup low-fat milk

SNACK

Spinach and Artichoke Heart Dip (page 261) with small baked whole wheat pita

- ◆ 1 serving dip, 1 pita

- ■ 1½ servings dip, 1 pita

- ● ½ to 1 serving dip, ½ to 1 pita

Fun Fruit Kebabs (page 263) dipped in low-fat vanilla yogurt

♦ 1 kebab, ½ cup yogurt

■ 1 kebab, ½ cup yogurt mixed with ¼ cup cottage cheese

● ½ to 1 kebab, ¼ to ½ cup yogurt

Popcorn, turkey slices with fresh tomatoes sprinkled with lemon pepper

♦ 3 cups popcorn, 1 ounce turkey, tomatoes

■ 3 cups popcorn, 2 ounces turkey, tomatoes

● 1 cup popcorn, ½ ounce turkey, tomatoes

LUNCH (EAT IN)

Sweet Potato Minestrone (page 246), grilled chicken

♦ 1 serving soup, 2 ounces chicken

■ 1 serving soup, 3 ounces chicken

● ½ serving soup, 1 to 2 ounces chicken

Zesty Tuna Salad (page 242) over whole wheat angel hair pasta, small apple

♦ ½ serving tuna salad, ½ cup pasta, 1 apple

■ ½ serving tuna salad, 1 cup pasta, 1 apple

● ¼ to ½ serving tuna salad, ¼ to ½ cup pasta, ½ apple

LUNCH (EAT OUT)

Taco Bell chicken enchirito "Fresco style"

♦ 1 enchirito

■ 1 enchirito

● ¼ to ½ enchirito

SNACK

Hard-cooked egg on whole grain toast

♦ 1 egg, 1 slice toast

■ 1 egg and 1 egg white, 1 slice toast

● ½ egg, ½ slice toast

Celery with thinly spread peanut butter topped with raisins

♦ 1 rib celery, 1 teaspoon peanut butter, 1 tablespoon raisins

■ 1 rib celery, 1 teaspoon peanut butter, 1 tablespoon raisins, 1 ounce turkey

● ½ to 1 rib celery, ½ to 1 teaspoon peanut butter, ½ to 1 tablespoon raisins

Low-fat cottage cheese with fresh cherries

♦ ¼ cup cottage cheese, ½ cup cherries

■ ½ cup cottage cheese, ½ cup cherries

● 2 to 3 tablespoons cottage cheese, ¼ cup cherries

DINNER

Grilled Beef Tenderloin (page 249), baked potato with low-fat sour cream, Roasted Asparagus (page 258), milk

♦ ½ serving beef, 1 small potato with 1 tablespoon sour cream, 1 serving asparagus, 1 cup fat-free milk

- ■ ½ serving beef, 1 large potato with 1 tablespoon sour cream, 1 serving asparagus, 1 cup fat-free milk

- ● ¼ serving beef, ½ small potato with ½ tablespoon sour cream, ½ serving asparagus, ½ to 1 cup low-fat milk

Soft tacos made with whole wheat tortillas, grilled steak or chicken, tomatoes, lettuce, grilled peppers, and low-fat cheese; milk

- ◆ 2 tortillas, 3 ounces meat, tomatoes, lettuce, and peppers, 1 ounce cheese, 1 cup fat-free milk

- ■ 3 tortillas, 4 ounces meat, tomatoes, lettuce, and peppers, 1 ounce cheese, 1 cup fat-free milk

- ● 1 tortilla, 1 to 2 ounces meat, tomatoes, lettuce, and peppers, ½ to 1 ounce cheese, ½ to 1 cup low-fat milk

Sloppy Joes (page 252) on whole grain bun, Baked French Fries (page 255), steamed carrots

- ◆ 1 bun, 1 serving Sloppy Joes, 1 serving fries, carrots

- ■ 1 bun, 1 serving Sloppy Joes, 1½ servings fries, carrots

- ● ½ bun, ¼ to ½ serving Sloppy Joes, ½ serving fries, carrots

▼ SUNDAY

Choose one option for each meal and snack.

BREAKFAST

Shrimp and Veggie Omelet (page 240) with whole grain toast

- ◆ 1 serving omelet, 1 slice toast

- ■ 1 serving omelet, 1 slice toast

- ● ¼ to ½ serving omelet, ½ to 1 slice toast

French toast made with whole grain bread, low-fat or vegetarian sausage

- ◆ 2 slices French toast, 1 piece sausage

- ■ 3 slices French toast, 2 pieces sausage

- ● ½ to 1 slice French toast, 1 piece sausage

Oatmeal with milk

- ◆ ½ cup oatmeal, 1 tablespoon protein powder, 1 cup fat-free milk

- ■ 1 cup oatmeal, 2 tablespoons protein powder, 1 cup fat-free milk

- ● ½ to 1 cup oatmeal, ½ to 1 cup low-fat milk

SNACK

One-half peanut butter and jelly sandwich on whole grain bread with sliced strawberries (with natural peanut butter and all-fruit jam)

- ◆ ½ slice bread, ½ teaspoon peanut butter, ½ teaspoon jam, ½ cup strawberries

- ■ 1 slice bread, 1 teaspoon peanut butter, 1 teaspoon jam, ½ cup strawberries

- ● ½ slice bread, ½ teaspoon peanut butter, ½ teaspoon jam, ¼ cup strawberries

Apple Ladybug Treats (page 260)

- ◆ 1 serving treats, 1 ounce ham

- ■ 1 serving treats, 2 ounces ham

- ● 1 serving treats

Reduced-fat mozzarella sticks and fresh pear

- ◆ 1 cheese stick, 1 pear

- ■ 2 cheese sticks, 1 pear

- ● ½ cheese stick, ½ pear

LUNCH (EAT IN)

Chicken Salad (page 244) on whole grain bread, red grapes

- ◆ 1 slice bread, 1 serving chicken salad, 15 grapes

- ■ 1 slice bread, 1 serving chicken salad, 15 grapes

- ● ½ to 1 slice bread, ¼ to ½ serving chicken salad, 6 to 10 grapes

Roast beef sandwich on whole grain bread, side salad with olive oil vinaigrette, cantaloupe cubes

- ◆ 1 slice bread, 2 ounces roast beef, 1 cup salad with 1 teaspoon olive oil and balsamic vinegar, 1 cup cantaloupe cubes

- ■ 2 slices bread, 3 ounces roast beef, 1 cup salad with 1 teaspoon olive oil and balsamic vinegar, 1 cup cantaloupe cubes

- ● ½ to 1 slice bread, 1 to 2 ounces roast beef, ¼ to ½ cup salad with ½ to 1 teaspoon olive oil and balsamic vinegar, ¼ to ½ cup cantaloupe cubes

LUNCH (EAT OUT)

Boston Market rotisserie turkey, steamed vegetable medley, butternut squash

- ◆ 2 ounces turkey, 1 cup vegetables, ½ cup squash

- ■ 3 ounces turkey, 1 cup vegetables, 1 cup squash

- ● 1 to 2 ounces turkey, ¼ to ½ cup vegetables, ¼ cup squash

SNACK

Low-fat vanilla yogurt mixed with frozen blueberries and sprinkled with sunflower seeds

- ◆ ½ cup yogurt, ½ cup blueberries, 1 tablespoon sunflower seeds

- ■ 1 cup yogurt, ½ cup blueberries, 1 tablespoon sunflower seeds

- ● ¼ to ½ cup yogurt, ¼ to ½ cup blueberries, 1 teaspoon sunflower seeds

Fruit Smoothie (page 263)

- ◆ ½ serving smoothie

- 1 serving smoothie, 2 tablespoons protein powder
- ¼ serving smoothie

Trail mix made with Wheat Chex, raisins, and peanuts or almonds

- ◆ ¼ cup Wheat Chex, 1 tablespoon raisins, ½ tablespoon nuts
- ■ ½ cup Wheat Chex, 2 tablespoons raisins, 1 tablespoon nuts
- ● ¼ to ½ cup Wheat Chex, ½ to 1 tablespoon raisins, ½ tablespoon nuts

DINNER

Chicken Creole (page 250), side salad with olive oil vinaigrette, milk

- ◆ 1 serving creole, 1 cup salad with 1 teaspoon olive oil and balsamic vinegar, 1 cup fat-free milk
- ■ 1 serving creole, 1 cup salad with 1 teaspoon olive oil and balsamic vinegar, 1 cup fat-free milk

- ● ¼ to ½ serving creole, ¼ to ½ cup salad with ½ to 1 teaspoon olive oil and balsamic vinegar, ½ to 1 cup low-fat milk

Baked Fish with Vegetables (page 250), whole wheat rotini with freshly grated Parmesan cheese

- ◆ 1 serving fish with vegetables, ½ cup rotini, 1 ounce cheese
- ■ 1 serving fish with vegetables, 1 cup rotini, 1 ounce cheese
- ● ½ serving fish with vegetables, ¼ cup rotini, ½ to 1 ounce cheese

Grilled lean steak, Roasted Vegetables (page 258), red potatoes

- ◆ 3 ounces steak, 1 serving vegetables, 1 cup potatoes
- ■ 4 ounces steak, 1 serving vegetables, 1½ cups potatoes
- ● 2 to 3 ounces steak, ½ to 1 serving vegetables, ½ to 1 cup potatoes

FITNESS FOCUS

Before we get into this week's topic, I want to remind you that the start of Week 4, the halfway point in our plan, is also a good time to check exercise habits that are forming or not forming. One healthy habit you want to make sure that you're forming is the journaling of dates and the time spent on activities. I also like the habit of putting the journal up in a central location for everyone to access.

It's not so hard, really—just remember to jot it down, and don't forget to set up a balanced reward system for you and your family. Try not to use food as part of the reward system. Instead, use nonfood items such as going to a sporting event or movie or buying new shoes, a new sport coat, or a baseball glove.

Week 4: Flexibility through Stretching

For our Week 4 Fitness Focus, we will add one of the most important elements of staying fit, preventing injuries, and maintaining good posture. It's called flexibility.

After you add just a few more minutes to your activity time, your program will include the keys to health and fitness: cardiovascular activity, strength training, core development, and now, flexibility through stretching. When practiced in concert, these four elements totally balance the body and allow it to function at its optimum levels. Your heart becomes stronger; your muscles and joints function properly; your core is protected from injury; and your body is long, lean, and relaxed.

Stretching your muscles can be one of the best things you do for your body. In fact, the older you get, the more focused and consistent you should be with your flexibility exercises. Stretching is for everyone, so start early and continue well into your golden years.

 SENA SAYS:
Everyone needs to stretch for good health at every age.

Let me show you how easy it is to put stretching into your lives and activity times. First, I recommend the same safe, easy-to-do stretches for children and adults of all ages.

The following 12 stretches can either be done all together at the end of your strength-training circuit or one at a time throughout the circuit. Doing your stretches in between your strength-training exercises keeps your muscles stretched and flexible throughout your workout and puts your rest time between strength exercises to good use. It also assures that you will get the stretches in and won't conveniently forget them because you are tired or pressed for time. On the other hand, doing the stretches at the end gives you a nice cooling-down period, relaxes your body, and lets your heart rate come down gradually. I advise my clients to alternate approaches. Both are effective, and it helps to change your routine so that you don't get bored with your fitness program.

Simply do the stretches on the following pages in order from 1 to 12.

❑ For adults (age 18 and older), stretch 3 days per week.

❑ For teenagers (ages 13 to 17), stretch 3 days per week.

❑ For children (age 12 and younger), stretch 2 days per week.

#1 STRAIGHT ARMS BEHIND BACK
(SHOULDERS, CHEST)

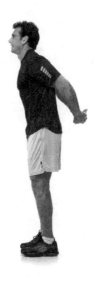

Here's how: Standing, place both arms behind your back. Interlock your fingers with your palms facing each other. Extend your elbows fully, then slowly raise your arms, keeping your elbows straight. Keep your head upright and neck relaxed. Hold for 30 seconds and release.

#2 CHICKEN WING
(TRICEPS, SHOULDERS, BACK)

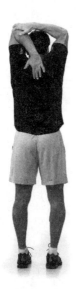

Here's how: Standing or sitting, raise your left arm and bend it at the elbow. Reach down toward your right shoulder blade; grasping your elbow with the other hand to increase the shoulder stretch. Hold for 30 seconds and release. Repeat with both arms.

#3 LOOK RIGHT AND LEFT

(NECK)

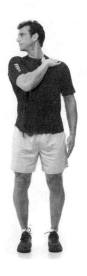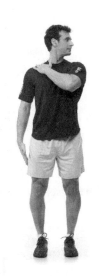

Here's how: Stand or sit with your head and neck in neutral position. Place your right hand on the top of your left shoulder while you slowly and gently look right. Keep your shoulders square and breathe normally. Hold for 30 seconds and then release. Repeat on the opposite side.

#4 NECK FLEXION

(NECK)

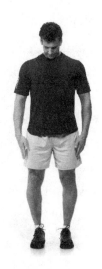

Here's how: Stand or sit with your head and neck in neutral position. With your eyes open, slowly and gently tuck your chin down toward your chest as far as you can and pause. Breathe normally. Hold for 30 seconds and then release.

#5 CROSS ARM OVER CHEST
(TRICEPS, SHOULDERS, UPPER BACK)

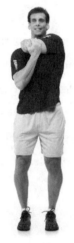

Here's how: While standing or sitting, bend your left elbow to 90 degrees. Place your right hand just above your elbow at your triceps and slowly and gently pull your left elbow across your body just beneath your chin line. Breathe normally. Hold for 30 seconds and then release. Repeat on the opposite side.

#6 SPINAL TWIST PRETZEL
(UPPER BACK, LOWER BACK, HIPS)

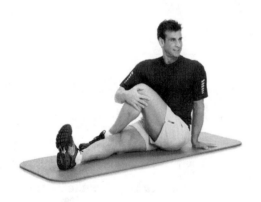

Here's how: Sit upright with good posture—chest up, shoulders back, and abdomen firm. Place your left foot flat on the floor on the outside of your right knee. (If this is difficult, place the foot on the inside of the knee.) Place your right hand on the outside of your left knee and your left arm straight down behind your hips. Slowly and gently pull your left knee over toward the right side while turning your head, neck, and torso toward the left. Breathe normally. Hold for 30 seconds and then release. Repeat on the opposite side.

#7 SUPINE KNEE FLEXION

(HIPS, BUTTOCKS, HAMSTRINGS)

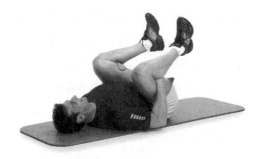

Here's how: Lie on your back and place both hands on the backs of your thighs just below your knees. With your eyes open, head, neck, shoulders, back, and hips flat, slowly and gently pull your knees toward your armpits. (For maximum stretch, keep your thighs to the sides of your torso as much as possible.) Pull down as firmly as possible without allowing your hips and lower back to lift up. Breathe normally. Hold for 30 seconds and then release.

#8 SIDE BEND WITH EXTENDED ARM

(OBLIQUES, BACK, ABDOMINALS)

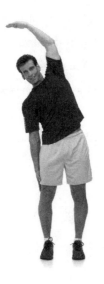

Here's how: Stand with your feet approximately 6 inches apart with proper posture—head and neck neutral, chest up, and shoulders, back, and knees slightly bent. Reach upward with your left arm, while your right arm stays at your side. Slowly and gently lean over to the right side as far as you can, while you continue to extend your left arm overhead. Breathe normally. Hold for 30 seconds and then release. Repeat on the opposite side.

#9 SIDE QUADRICEPS STRETCH
(QUADRICEPS, HIP FLEXORS)

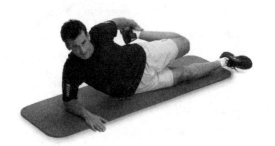

Here's how: Lie on your right side with both legs straight. Place your right fore-arm and the palm of your hand flat on the floor, keeping your elbow underneath your shoulder. Grasp the front of your left ankle with your left hand and slowly and gently pull your heel toward your buttocks. Breathe normally. Hold for 30 seconds and release. Repeat on the opposite side.

#10 SUPINE HAMSTRING STRETCH
(HAMSTRINGS, LUMBAR, CALVES)

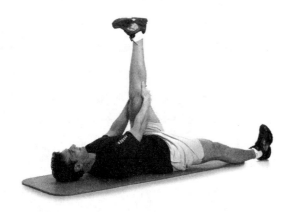

Here's how: Lie on the floor with both legs straight. Slowly and gently raise one leg and grasp it behind the knee with both hands. Your other leg should be as straight as possible, but a slight bend is okay. Breathe normally. Hold for 30 seconds and then release. Repeat with other leg.

#11 STANDING STRETCH
(CALVES, ACHILLES TENDONS)

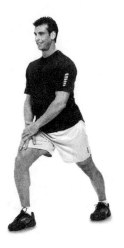

Here's how: Place either foot forward and step back with the other leg. Place both hands on top of the front thigh while leaning forward and keeping your back flat. The heel of the back foot should be flat on the floor at all times. Breathe normally. Hold for 30 seconds and then release. Repeat with opposite leg.

#12 CHILD'S POSE
(SHOULDERS, BACK, HIPS)

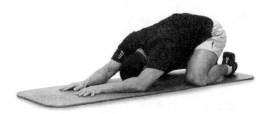

Here's how: Start in a kneeling position with your knees shoulder width apart and pointing slightly outward. Slowly and gently sit back on your heels. Continue to lower your body toward the floor as you reach forward with your hands. Breathe slowly and deeply as you allow your body to relax and get as close to the floor as possible. Hold for 30 seconds and then release.

Once again, let's use a convenient grid to help you visualize how easily these activities now fit into your weekly schedules without eating up your day! *Note:* In my example in the grid, Sunday is called family day. Although I want everyone to try to have 1 day of rest each week, the family can either choose Sunday for their Fit Family Activity or do it on another day (which counts toward everyone's weekly activity).

	M	T	W	TH	F	S	SU
Children 12 and younger	C:30 min	ST:12 min + F:6	C:30 min	ST:12 min + F:6	C:30 min	C:30 min	F A M I L Y D A Y
Teenagers 13 to 17	C:30 min	ST:12 min + F:6	C:30 min	ST:12 min + F:6	C:30 min	C:30 min + ST:12 + F:6	
Adults 18 and older	C:30 min + ST:12 + F:6	C:30 min	ST:12 min + F:6	C:30 min	C:30 min	ST:12 min + F:6	

KEY: C = Cardio activities; ST = Strength training + core; F = flexibility
Note: These days were selected for example purposes. You can copy this schedule or have everyone select their own.

As you can see, we've added only 6 minutes per day to our strength-training sessions, which now include core movements and stretching. In just 4 weeks, you and your family have adopted a totally well-balanced fitness program that will fit into your schedules very easily. That's why this 6-week program works—it's doable for the entire family!

FIT FAMILY ACTIVITY

Go take a hike! How many times have we heard that from someone in our lives? But hiking is actually a great form of exercise, and it can be a lot of fun.

Hiking utilizes most of the body's muscles and can be challenging, depending on the terrain. I like using a hiking stick for more upper-body involvement and to push away brush if needed. Most important, you'll use many of your ankle, knee, and hip stabilizing muscles, and you will feel the challenge. It can also turn into fun by offering opportunities to climb rocks and trees, hop over streams, and roll down hills. You can do some rock collecting or count the different species of birds while you and your family have a picnic. On flat terrain, you can have three-legged races or wheelbarrow races for something different. Use your imagination and watch what happens. When hiking, you always want to practice safety, and make sure that you take plenty of water, healthy snacks, and a first-aid kit with you.

If it's too cold or rainy for a hike, take a family trip down to your neighborhood bowling alley. It's fun and helps improve balance, agility, and hand/eye coordination. The family competition is always great, and everyone always has a good time. Just watch out for the unhealthy food and beverage choices everywhere. I suggest that you pack some healthy sandwiches and some 100% pure fruit juice. (For more outdoor and indoor activity ideas, see appendix B.)

You are really making it happen! Good job. Mom, keep it going . . .

WEEK 4 FINAL THOUGHTS

I want you and your family to know that you are doing a great job. I know that I've given you a lot to digest in these 4 weeks, but as you follow my suggestions, I promise that you will begin to feel that you are on the path to health. I leave you with this advice that a wise old man once gave me. "To be successful, you simply have to form the habits and embrace doing the things that failures just won't do." Here's to a healthy and successful week!

WEEK 4 ACTION STEP SUMMARY

❑ Hold your Week 4 Fit Family Meeting.
❑ Acknowledge and congratulate your family for hitting the halfway point.
❑ Take the Fit Family Quiz again and see how far you've come.
❑ Review your food diaries and exercise/activity journals and root out any lapses.
❑ Make fun part of the process.
❑ Plan your week's healthy meals, focusing on fruits and veggies.
❑ Integrate flexibility exercises into your weekly program.
❑ Plan your Fit Family Activity: take a vigorous family hike or go bowling.
❑ Schedule your Week 5 Fit Family Meeting.

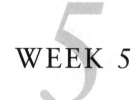

Boost Your Metabolism with Healthy Snacks

With only 2 weeks left in your plan, your family should really be shifting into high gear! This is the home stretch—a perfect time to plan and prioritize your remaining challenges. In other words, tally up what's working and be honest about your trouble spots and the areas that have been a challenge for each member of your family.

JUST FOR YOU, MOM

Hey, Coach; it's our time to talk again—just you and me. After taking on a healthy lifestyle and exercising, most people start to see a lot of benefits. You should too. By now, Mom, you should be:

   1. Feeling better and stronger because you are doing something positive and good for yourself. You will also feel mentally stronger because of your increased brain power as a result of eating healthier foods. Foods that contain high amounts of fat and sugar make us mentally lethargic. As you pull foods like these out of your daily menus, your improved mental clarity will soon be obvious.

2. Experiencing an emotional lift from exercise as endorphins help dissipate feelings of anxiety and even depression during the course of your day.

3. Starting to look and feel different, first in your clothes and then in the mirror. In other words, as you tone your muscles and start shrinking unwanted fat cells, your overall appearance will drastically change not only to *your* eyes but also to everyone else who sees you.

You will lose weight this week, Mom, if you:

❏ Incorporate my interval-training techniques into your exercise routines (burns calories and improves athletic abilities).

❏ Bring your overall workout intensity up another notch on the R.P.E. scale (continues to increase fat-burning efficiency).

❏ Cut back on sugar from desserts by half (stabilizes blood sugar and curbs cravings).

SENA SAYS:
Now is the time to make final adjustments that will guide you toward "mission accomplished."

❏ Eliminate two of these items for a week: alcohol; white bread, rice and pasta; creamy gravy; full-fat salad dressing; processed foods (boosts weight loss).

WEEK 5 FIT FAMILY MEETING AGENDA

❏ Make adjustments to your strategies where needed.

❏ Review food diaries and red flag any saturated fat or sugar lapses.

❏ Review exercise/activity journals—are family members sticking with their routines?

❏ Plan a new week of healthy menus—Food Focus: snacks and desserts

❏ Discuss your Week 5 Fitness Focus: Michael's personal interval-training routines

❏ Plan your Fit Family Activity: Have a ball!

❏ Schedule your Week 6 Fit Family Meeting.

WEEK 5 FIT FAMILY MEETING

As my "sideline coach," I'm asking you to help each member of your family build on their strengths and, more important, to focus on the areas where progress has been slow. Start by keeping your sense of fun and enthusiasm high and by letting everyone know how proud you are of them. (I'm sure that they are proud of you too.) Each of the next 14 days will provide an opportunity to capitalize on the past month of hard work.

REVIEW YOUR FOOD DIARIES

Since you're getting close to being a "graduate" of my program, I'm going to give you two assignments this week when reviewing your food diaries.

Assignment 1: How did your family members do with limiting saturated and hydrogenated fat in their meal plans? Check your food diaries and use a yellow highlighter to mark items such as fried foods, high-fat meats, pastries and doughnuts, pies and cakes, butter or regular margarine, and snack foods with hydrogenated fats—including cheese, butter, crackers, cookies, and chips. Next, take a blue highlighter and look for foods with healthy unsaturated fats, such as avocados, fatty fish, nuts, and olive oil. If you see a lot more yellow than blue, you have some work to do!

Set a goal to *decrease* the amount of foods containing bad fats by one serving per day over the next week. In addition, focus on eating healthy fats for the fat servings in your meal plan. For example, add a small slice of avocado to your salad or sandwich, make a trail mix with almonds and raisins for a snack, or sprinkle sunflower seeds in your cottage cheese. While you're at it, check to make sure that the portions of these healthy fats are the size they should be. The following are each equal to one serving of fat.

❏ 1 teaspoon oil
❏ 8 almonds, walnuts, or pecans
❏ 1 tablespoon peanuts (about 6 to 8)

❏ 1 tablespoon sunflower seeds
❏ 2 teaspoons natural peanut butter
❏ ⅛ avocado

As I mentioned earlier, by limiting the bad fats and concentrating on good fats, you are decreasing your risk of heart disease and gaining numerous additional health benefits.

Assignment 2: For your second "assignment," I'd like to ask you to go through your diaries and circle those foods you have eaten that are high in sugar (such as candy, ice cream, cookies, soda, and chocolate). Evaluate how often you are eating them. If you eat in moderation (a small amount every couple of days), then it's okay if they are foods you really enjoy. However, if you indulge more often, such as every day or several times a day, then you are most likely setting yourself up to fail. Eating high-sugar foods will cause you to crave more of them, which will result either in eating too many calories or in displacing healthy calories. If you're eating too many sweets, set a goal to decrease your sugary food intake by one serving per day over the next week.

After reviewing your food diaries, did you find that there was room for improvement in your family's relationship with "the bad guys"—saturated fats and sugar? If so, you'll want to pay special attention to this week's Food Focus.

WEEK 5 FOOD FOCUS: SNACKS AND DESSERTS

This week, I have two different Food Focus topics I would like to discuss with you. The first one is healthy snacks, an extremely important part of your daily meal plan. Small snacks that include lean protein and fiber are vital to prevent your blood sugar from dropping between meals, which will lead to overeating. The second topic is one that is not so vital to my meal plan, but it's something that is important to most of us—desserts! Instead of completely banishing desserts from our meal plans, which we all know is unrealistic, I'm going to give you some suggestions for low-calorie and low-fat treats and recommendations on how to include them so that you can continue to reach your goals.

Healthy Snacks

As you know, small, frequent meals are a large part of this meal program, so snacks are obviously very important. As part of your cupboard cleaning, you should have rid your shelves of all of the junky snack temptations, but some of you may be holding on to your favorites. Plus, the corner store and vending machines are still accessible. Some of your food diaries may have revealed that you're having a hard time giving up high-sugar, high-fat, low-nutrient snacks such as candy, chips, cheesy crackers, granola bars, or high-sugar yogurt.

These foods are okay every once in a while, but the best way to avoid craving them is to eat lean protein and complex carbohydrates throughout the day. Often, we eat these snacks because we're not sure what kinds of healthy foods to eat instead. Check out the following list of snacks for some new ideas (see the meal plans for serving sizes that are appropriate for you).

HEALTHY SNACKS	UNHEALTHY SNACKS
Reduced-fat mozzarella sticks with fresh or dried fruit	High-sugar yogurt
Low-fat plain or vanilla yogurt mixed with fresh berries	Ice cream
Tuna salad on whole grain crackers or toast (try adding sliced grapes, celery, and onions for a crunchy, sweet flavor)	Cheese snack crackers
Natural peanut butter on an apple	Toaster pastries
Natural peanut butter spread on celery sticks with raisins	Fruit roll-ups or "fruity" snacks
Fresh veggies dipped in hummus or cottage cheese dip	Cheese curls
Edamame (buy it precooked and frozen; it heats up in only 2 minutes in the microwave)	Large amount of nuts
Trail mix with raisins, dried apricots, sunflower seeds, and pumpkin seeds	Trail mix with chocolate chips, candy pieces, and nuts
Hard-cooked egg sliced on a slice of whole grain toast	Cinnamon bun
Energy protein bar	Candy bar or high-fat granola bar
Toasted whole wheat pita triangles dipped in warm, fat-free refried beans with salsa	Tortilla chips dipped in nacho sauce
Fruit smoothie	Milkshake

It's important to plan your snacks ahead, since most of us are away from home at snack time. This may mean taking a bag of snacks to work at the beginning of the week to keep in the refrigerator or your desk drawer. Some people may prefer to pack their snacks along with their lunches each day. I try to always keep some nonperishable foods such as energy bars, trail mixes, or dried fruit in my car, my bag, or my desk drawer.

Of course, there will be days when you just don't have time to prepare something, or you haven't been to the grocery store in a while. If this happens, you have several options. You can choose something from the "eating out" lunch sections in Weeks 2 and 6 and have a smaller portion or save part of it for your next meal. Another option is to run into a convenience store and pick up an energy bar, piece of fruit, box of raisins, yogurt, or a sandwich (save half for later). The important thing is to not skip your meals and snacks if at all possible. Remember that this will only make you eat more at your next meal and can set you up for sugar or salt cravings.

Desserts

Mmmm . . . desserts . . . I *love* desserts. From my mom's homemade blueberry pie with vanilla ice cream to gooey, chocolate brownies, I truly enjoy the real deal. However, I believe I enjoy them because I have only a moderate serving two or three times a month. For some families, having a bowl of ice cream or a piece of pie after dinner every night is a very routine and sacred part of the day. Unfortunately, eating high-calorie, high-fat sweets every night is really going to work against your goals. For one thing, dessert provides extra calories, which add up to extra weight gained or difficulty losing the extra weight you already have. One cup of ice cream (½ pint) has 600 calories. One piece of cake with frosting has more than 400 calories, and a piece of fruit pie can have more than 350. In addition, all of the sugar you eat can actually cause you to crave more, and having sweets around the house is tempting for everyone. However, if dessert is really important to you and your family, you can include it in your meal plans once or twice a week. Here are my suggestions.

1. Eat moderate-size servings (no seconds!).

2. Choose lower-fat options by substituting low-fat yogurt, fruit puree, or applesauce for all or part of the oil in cake and brownie recipes.

3. Increase exercise to burn off the extra calories by doing an extra 20 minutes of cardio.

In addition, you can try some of these desserts that are lower in fat and calories.

❏ ½ cup frozen yogurt or low-fat ice cream

❏ ½ cup fruit sorbet or sherbet

❏ ½ cup Creamy Rice Pudding (page 265)

❏ ½ cup fruit crisp

❏ ½ cup Yummy Fruit Salad (page 265)

❏ 1 cup hot chocolate made with fat-free milk

❏ 3 or 4 small cookies

❏ 1 slice angel food cake with berries

❏ Vanilla Berry Parfaits (page 264)

❏ 1 slice fruit pie with graham cracker crust

❏ Baked Pears (page 264)

WEEK 5 MENU PLAN

◆ = goal weight 160 pounds or lower

■ = goal weight over 160 pounds

● = kids age 12 and under

▼ MONDAY

Choose one option for each meal and snack.

BREAKFAST

Oatmeal with milk

- ◆ ½ cup oatmeal, 1 tablespoon protein powder, 1 cup fat-free milk

- ■ 1 cup oatmeal, 2 tablespoons protein powder, 1 cup fat-free milk

- ● ½ to 1 cup oatmeal, ½ to 1 cup low-fat milk

Whole grain frozen waffles, vegetarian or low-fat sausage

- ◆ 2 waffles, 2 pieces sausage

- ■ 3 waffles, 3 pieces sausage

- ● 1 to 1½ waffles, 1 piece sausage

Breakfast Sandwich (page 237)

- ◆ 1 sandwich

- ■ 1 sandwich, 1 piece fruit

- ● ½ sandwich

SNACK

Reduced-fat mozzarella sticks with raisins

- ◆ 1 cheese stick, 2 tablespoons raisins

- ■ 2 cheese sticks, 2 tablespoons raisins

- ● ½ cheese stick, 1 tablespoon raisins

Thinly spread peanut butter on whole grain toast, apple

- ◆ ½ teaspoon peanut butter, ½ slice toast, ½ apple, 1 ounce turkey

- ■ 1 teaspoon peanut butter, 1 slice toast, 1 apple, 1 ounce turkey

- ● ½ teaspoon peanut butter, ¼ to ½ slice toast, ¼ to ½ apple

Fruit Smoothie (page 263)

- ◆ ½ serving smoothie

- ■ 1 serving smoothie, 2 tablespoons protein powder

- ● ¼ serving smoothie

LUNCH (EAT IN)

Chickpea Salad with Red Onion and Tomato (page 256), tuna

- ◆ 1 serving salad, 2 ounces tuna

- ■ 1½ servings salad, 3 ounces tuna

¼ to ½ serving salad, 1 to 2 ounces tuna

LUNCH (EAT OUT)

6" Subway turkey, ham, or roast beef sandwich on wheat bread with 1 added fat (either cheese, mayo, or oil)

♦ 1 sandwich with 1 added fat

■ 1 sandwich with 1 added fat

● ½ sandwich with 1 added fat

LUNCH (AT SCHOOL)

Turkey Apple Sandwich (page 243), baby carrots

♦ 1 sandwich, carrots

■ 1 sandwich, carrots

● ¼ to ½ sandwich, carrots

SNACK

Edamame (soybeans)—buy fresh or frozen and boil. If precooked, heat in microwave.

♦ ½ cup edamame

■ 1 cup edamame

● ¼ cup edamame

Low-fat cheese on whole grain crackers, grapes

♦ 1 ounce cheese, 4 crackers, 8 grapes

■ 2 ounces cheese, 4 crackers, 8 grapes

● ½ to 1 ounce cheese, 4 crackers, 6 to 10 grapes

Zesty Tuna Salad (page 242) on whole grain crackers, apple

♦ ¼ serving tuna, 3 crackers, ½ apple

■ ½ serving tuna, 6 crackers, ½ apple

● ¼ serving tuna, 2 or 3 crackers, ¼ apple

DINNER

Grilled tuna steaks, whole wheat angel hair pasta with steamed asparagus and carrots, sprinkled with freshly grated Parmesan cheese

♦ 3 ounces tuna, 1 cup pasta with vegetables, 1 ounce cheese

■ 4 ounces tuna, 1½ cups pasta with vegetables, 1 ounce cheese

● 1 to 2 ounces tuna, ¼ to ½ cup pasta with vegetables, ½ to 1 ounce cheese

Chicken Vegetable Stew (page 248), small whole grain roll, side salad with olive oil vinaigrette

♦ 1 serving stew, 1 roll, 1 cup salad with 1 teaspoon olive oil and balsamic vinegar

■ 1 serving stew, 1 roll, 1 cup salad with 1 teaspoon olive oil and balsamic vinegar

● ¼ to ½ serving stew, 1 roll, ¼ to ½ cup side salad with ½ teaspoon olive oil and balsamic vinegar

Lean beef hamburger on whole wheat bun, Coleslaw Salad (page 259)

♦ 1 bun, 3-ounce hamburger, 1 serving coleslaw

- 1 bun, 4-ounce hamburger, 1½ servings coleslaw

- ½ to 1 bun, 1- to 2-ounce hamburger, ¼ to ½ serving coleslaw

▼TUESDAY

Choose one option for each meal and snack.

BREAKFAST

High-fiber, high-protein cereal with milk

- ◆ ½ cup cereal, 3 tablespoons protein powder, 1 cup fat-free milk

- ■ 1 cup cereal, 3 tablespoons protein powder, 1 cup fat-free milk

- ● ½ to 1 cup cereal, ½ to 1 cup low-fat milk

Low-fat vanilla yogurt with fresh orange slices

- ◆ 1 cup yogurt, ½ orange

- ■ 1½ cups yogurt, 1 orange

- ● ½ to 1 cup yogurt, ¼ to ½ orange

Ham and Vegetable Frittata (page 238) with whole grain toast

- ◆ 1 serving frittata, 1 slice toast

- ■ 1½ servings frittata, 1 slice toast

- ● ½ serving frittata, ½ slice toast

SNACK

Protein bar (14+ grams protein, 25 grams carbohydrates, less than 3 grams fat)

- ◆ ½ energy bar

- ■ 1 energy bar

- ● ¼ to ½ energy bar

Fun Fruit Kebabs (page 263) dipped in low-fat yogurt

- ◆ 1 kebab, ½ cup yogurt

- ■ 1 kebab, ½ cup yogurt mixed with ¼ cup cottage cheese

- ● ½ to 1 kebab, ¼ to ½ cup yogurt

Veggie Dip (page 262) with fresh-cut vegetables

- ◆ 1 serving dip, veggies

- ■ 1 serving dip, veggies, 1 ounce turkey

- ● ½ to 1 serving dip, veggies

LUNCH (EAT IN)

Tomato soup, whole grain crackers, baby carrots

- ◆ 1 cup soup (made with fat-free milk), 6 crackers, carrots

- ■ 1½ cups soup (made with fat-free milk), 8 crackers, carrots

- ● ½ cup soup (made with low-fat milk), 3 to 6 crackers, carrots

LUNCH (EAT OUT)

Arby's roast beef wrap with light cheese and no sauce

- ◆ 1 wrap

- 1 wrap, 1 cup fat-free milk

- ¼ to ½ wrap

LUNCH (AT SCHOOL)

Turkey sandwich on whole grain bread with lettuce and tomato, grape tomatoes, red grapes

- ◆ 1 slice bread, 2 ounces turkey, lettuce and tomato, grape tomatoes, 15 grapes

- ■ 2 slices bread, 3 ounces turkey, lettuce and tomato, grape tomatoes, 15 grapes

- ● ½ to 1 slice bread, 1 ounce turkey, lettuce and tomato, grape tomatoes, 6 to 10 grapes

SNACK

Fresh Homemade Salsa (page 260) with baked chips

- ◆ Salsa, 6 chips

- ■ Salsa, 12 chips

- ● Salsa, 6 chips

Low-fat cottage cheese with fresh pineapple and almonds

- ◆ ¼ cup cottage cheese, ½ cup pineapple, 8 almonds

- ■ ½ cup cottage cheese, 1 cup pineapple, 8 almonds

- ● 2 to 3 tablespoons cottage cheese, ¼ cup pineapple, 3 to 4 almonds

Apple Ladybug Treats (page 260)

- ◆ 1 serving treats, 1 ounce ham

- ■ 1 serving treats, 2 ounces ham

- ● 1 serving treats

DINNER

Grilled Salmon (page 245), baked sweet potato, steamed broccoli and cauliflower

- ◆ 1 serving salmon, 1 small potato, broccoli and cauliflower

- ■ 1 serving salmon, 1 large potato, broccoli and cauliflower

- ● ½ serving salmon, ¼ to ½ small potato, broccoli and cauliflower

Asian Steak (page 253), brown rice

- ◆ 1 serving steak, ⅔ cup rice

- ■ 1 serving steak, ⅔ cup rice, 1 cup fat-free milk

- ● ¼ to ½ serving steak, ⅓ cup rice

Soft tacos made with whole wheat tortillas, lean grilled steak or chicken, tomatoes and lettuce, and low-fat cheese; milk

- ◆ 2 tortillas, 3 ounces meat, tomatoes and lettuce, 1 ounce cheese, 1 cup fat-free milk

- ■ 3 tortillas, 4 ounces meat, tomatoes and lettuce, 1 ounce cheese, 1 cup fat-free milk

- ● 1 tortilla, 1 to 2 ounces meat, tomatoes and lettuce, ½ to 1 ounce cheese, ½ to 1 cup low-fat milk

Choose one option for each meal and snack.

BREAKFAST

Low-fat cheese melted on small whole wheat bagel

- ◆ 2 ounces cheese, 1 bagel
- ■ 2 ounces cheese, 1 bagel, 1 cup fat-free milk
- ● 1 ounce cheese, ½ to 1 bagel

French toast made with whole grain bread, low-fat or vegetarian sausage

- ◆ 2 slices French toast, 1 piece sausage
- ■ 3 slices French toast, 2 pieces sausage
- ● ½ to 1 slice French toast, 1 piece sausage

Shrimp and Veggie Omelet (page 240) with whole grain toast

- ◆ 1 serving omelet, 1 slice toast
- ■ 1 serving omelet, 1 slice toast
- ● ¼ to ½ serving omelet, ½ to 1 slice toast

SNACK

Low-fat cottage cheese with fresh cherries

- ◆ ¼ cup cottage cheese, 6 cherries
- ■ ½ cup cottage cheese, 12 cherries
- ● 2 tablespoons cottage cheese, 4 to 6 cherries

Trail mix made with Wheat Chex, raisins, and peanuts or almonds

- ◆ ¼ cup Wheat Chex, 1 tablespoon raisins, ½ tablespoon nuts
- ■ ½ cup Wheat Chex, 2 tablespoons raisins, 1 tablespoon nuts
- ● ¼ to ½ cup Wheat Chex, ½ to 1 tablespoon raisins, ½ tablespoon nuts

Spiced Pumpkin Seeds (page 262) and raisins

- ◆ ¼ cup pumpkin seeds, 1 tablespoon raisins
- ■ ¼ cup pumpkin seeds, 2 tablespoons raisins
- ● 2 to 4 tablespoons pumpkin seeds, 1 tablespoon raisins

LUNCH (EAT IN)

Chili made with lean beef, kidney beans, diced carrots, and green peppers; fresh orange slices

- ◆ 2 ounces beef, ½ cup beans, carrots, and green peppers, 1 orange
- ■ 3 ounces beef, 1 cup beans, carrots, and green peppers, 1 orange
- ● 1 to 2 ounces beef, ¼ to ½ cup beans, carrots, and green peppers, ¼ to ½ orange

LUNCH (EAT OUT)

Taco Bell steak enchirito "Fresco style"

- ◆ ½ enchirito

- ■ 1 enchirito

- ● ¼ to ½ enchirito

LUNCH (AT SCHOOL)

Vegetable Sandwich (page 243)

- ◆ 1 sandwich

- ■ 1 sandwich, 1 cup fat-free milk

- ● ½ sandwich

SNACK

Hummus and fresh vegetables

- ◆ 4 tablespoons hummus, vegetables

- ■ 6 tablespoons hummus, vegetables

- ● 2 tablespoons hummus, vegetables

Celery with thinly spread peanut butter topped with raisins

- ◆ 1 rib celery, 1 teaspoon peanut butter, 1 tablespoon raisins

- ■ 1 rib celery, 1 teaspoon peanut butter, 1 tablespoon raisins, 1 ounce turkey

- ● ½ to 1 rib celery, ½ to 1 teaspoon peanut butter, ½ to 1 tablespoon raisins

Reduced-fat mozzarella sticks and fresh pear

- ◆ 1 cheese stick, 1 pear

- ■ 2 cheese sticks, 1 pear

- ● ½ cheese stick, ½ pear

DINNER

Chicken Creole (page 250), side salad with olive oil vinaigrette, milk

- ◆ 1 serving creole, 1 cup salad with 1 teaspoon olive oil and balsamic vinegar, 1 cup fat-free milk

- ■ 1 serving creole, 1 cup salad with 1 teaspoon olive oil and balsamic vinegar, 1 cup fat-free milk

- ● ¼ to ½ serving creole, ¼ to ½ cup salad with ½ to 1 teaspoon olive oil and balsamic vinegar, ½ to 1 cup low-fat milk

Baked Fish with Vegetables (page 250), whole wheat rotini with freshly grated Parmesan cheese

- ◆ 1 serving fish with vegetables, ½ cup rotini, 1 ounce cheese

- ■ 1 serving fish with vegetables, 1 cup rotini, 1 ounce cheese

- ● ½ serving fish with vegetables, ¼ cup rotini, ½ to 1 ounce cheese

Grilled lean steak, Roasted Vegetables (page 258), red potatoes, milk

- ◆ 3 ounces steak, 1 serving vegetables, 1 cup potatoes, 1 cup fat-free milk

- ■ 4 ounces steak, 1 serving vegetables, 1½ cups potatoes, 1 cup fat-free milk

- ● 2 to 3 ounces steak, ½ to 1 serving vegetables, ½ to 1 cup potatoes, ½ to 1 cup low-fat milk

Choose one option for each meal and snack.

BREAKFAST

Oatmeal with milk

◆ ½ cup oatmeal, 1 tablespoon protein powder, 1 cup fat-free milk

■ 1 cup oatmeal, 2 tablespoons protein powder, 1 cup fat-free milk

● ½ to 1 cup oatmeal, ½ to 1 cup low-fat milk

Whole Wheat Pancakes (page 239), vegetarian or low-fat sausage

◆ 2 pancakes, 2 pieces sausage

■ 3 pancakes, 3 pieces sausage

● 1 or 2 pancakes, 1 or 2 pieces sausage

Breakfast Sandwich (page 237)

◆ 1 sandwich

■ 1 sandwich, 1 piece fruit

● ½ sandwich

SNACK

Apple Ladybug Treats (page 260)

◆ 1 serving treats, 1 ounce turkey

■ 1 serving treats, 2 ounces turkey

● 1 serving treats

Turkey and low-fat cheese slices, whole grain crackers, dried apricots

◆ ½ ounce turkey, ½ ounce cheese, 3 crackers, 2 apricots

■ 1 ounce turkey, 1 ounce cheese, 6 crackers, 4 apricots

● ½ ounce turkey, ½ ounce cheese, 2 or 3 crackers, 1 apricot

Low-fat cottage cheese with fresh pineapple

◆ ¼ cup cottage cheese, ½ cup pineapple

■ ½ cup cottage cheese, 1 cup pineapple

● 2 to 3 tablespoons cottage cheese, ¼ cup pineapple

LUNCH (EAT IN)

Wild Rice Apple Salad (page 255), grilled chicken

◆ ½ serving salad, 2 ounces chicken

■ 1 serving salad, 3 ounces chicken

● ¼ serving salad, 1 ounce chicken

LUNCH (EAT OUT)

McDonald's grilled chicken Caesar salad with low-fat dressing, apple slices

◆ 1 salad with 1 tablespoon dressing, 1 apple

■ 1 salad with 1 tablespoon dressing, 1 apple

● ½ to 1 salad with ½ tablespoon dressing, ½ to 1 apple

LUNCH (AT SCHOOL)

Low-fat cheese and tomato sandwich on whole wheat pita with Dijon mustard; apple slices; baby carrots

- ◆ 1 pita, 2 ounces cheese, tomato slices, 1 apple, carrots

- ■ 1 pita, 2 ounces cheese, tomato slices, 1 apple, carrots, 1 cup fat-free milk

- ● ½ to 1 pita, 1 to 2 ounces cheese, tomato slices, ¼ to ½ apple, carrots

SNACK

Veggie Dip (page 262) with fresh-cut vegetables

- ◆ 1 serving dip, vegetables

- ■ 2 servings dip, vegetables

- ● ½ serving dip, vegetables

Low-fat cottage cheese mixed with low-fat sour cream and sprinkled with cinnamon and brown sugar, with fresh fruit for dipping

- ◆ ¼ cup cottage cheese, 1 tablespoon sour cream, ½ cup fruit

- ■ ½ cup cottage cheese, 1 tablespoon sour cream, ½ cup fruit

- ● 2 to 3 tablespoons cottage cheese, ½ tablespoon sour cream, ¼ cup fruit

Hard-cooked egg on whole grain toast

- ◆ 1 egg, 1 slice toast

- ■ 1 egg and 1 egg white, 1 slice toast

- ● ½ egg, ½ slice toast

DINNER

Veggie burger on whole grain bun with lettuce and tomato, Baked French Fries made with sweet potatoes (page 255), broccoli sprinkled with low-fat cheese

- ◆ 1 bun, 1 burger, lettuce and tomato, ½ serving fries, broccoli with 1 ounce cheese

- ■ 1 bun, 1 burger, lettuce and tomato, 1 serving fries, broccoli with 1 ounce cheese

- ● ½ bun, ¼ to ½ burger, lettuce and tomato, ¼ to ½ serving fries, broccoli with ½ to 1 ounce cheese

Black Bean Soup (page 248); sliced tomato, fresh mozzarella, and basil salad sprinkled with balsamic vinaigrette; milk

- ◆ 1 serving soup, tomatoes with ½ ounce cheese and basil, 1 cup fat-free milk

- ■ 1 serving soup, tomatoes with 1 ounce cheese and basil, 1 cup fat-free milk

- ● ¼ to ½ serving soup, tomatoes with ½ ounce cheese and basil, ½ to 1 cup low-fat milk

Cabbage Roll-Ups (page 249), side salad with olive oil vinaigrette, milk

- ◆ 1 serving roll-ups, 1 cup salad with 1 teaspoon olive oil and balsamic vinegar, 1 cup fat-free milk

■ 1½ servings roll-ups, 1 cup salad with 1 teaspoon olive oil and balsamic vinegar, 1 cup fat-free milk

● ¼ to ½ serving roll-ups, ¼ to ½ cup salad with ½ teaspoon olive oil and balsamic vinegar, ½ to 1 cup low-fat milk

▼FRIDAY

Choose one option for each meal and snack.

BREAKFAST

High-fiber, high-protein cereal with milk

◆ ½ cup cereal, 3 tablespoons protein powder, 1 cup fat-free milk

■ 1 cup cereal, 3 tablespoons protein powder, 1 cup fat-free milk

● ½ to 1 cup cereal, ½ to 1 cup low-fat milk

Scrambled egg with whole grain toast

◆ 1 egg and 1 egg white, 2 slices toast

■ 1 egg and 2 egg whites, 3 slices toast

● 1 egg, 1 slice toast

Low-fat vanilla yogurt with sliced fresh strawberries

◆ 1 cup yogurt, ½ cup strawberries

■ 1½ cups yogurt, 1 cup strawberries

● ½ to 1 cup yogurt, ¼ to ½ cup strawberries

SNACK

Popcorn sprinkled with grated Parmesan cheese

◆ 3 cups popcorn, 1 ounce cheese

■ 3 cups popcorn, 1 ounce cheese

● 1 cup popcorn, ½ to 1 ounce cheese

Apple slices with thinly spread peanut butter

◆ 1 apple, 2 teaspoons peanut butter

■ 1 apple, 2 teaspoons peanut butter

● ¼ to ½ apple, 1 teaspoon peanut butter

Low-fat vanilla yogurt mixed with frozen blueberries and sprinkled with sunflower seeds

◆ ½ cup yogurt, ½ cup blueberries, 1 tablespoon sunflower seeds

■ 1 cup yogurt, ½ cup blueberries, 1 tablespoon sunflower seeds

● ¼ to ½ cup yogurt, ¼ to ½ cup blueberries, 1 teaspoon sunflower seeds

LUNCH (EAT IN)

Split pea soup made with ham, carrots, celery, and onions; small whole grain roll; milk

◆ 1 cup soup (with 1 ounce ham), 1 roll, 1 cup fat-free milk

■ 1½ cups soup (with 2 ounces ham), 1 roll, 1 cup fat-free milk

● ½ to ¾ cup soup (with ½ to 1 ounce ham), ½ roll, ½ to 1 cup low-fat milk

LUNCH (EAT OUT)

6" Subway turkey and ham sandwich wrap with 1 added fat (either cheese, mayo, or oil), grapes

- ◆ 1 wrap with 1 added fat, 15 grapes
- ■ 1 wrap with 1 added fat, 15 grapes, 1 cup fat-free milk
- ● ½ wrap with 1 added fat, 6 to 10 grapes

LUNCH (AT SCHOOL)

Peanut butter and jelly sandwich on medium (4" diameter) whole grain bagel (with natural peanut butter and all-fruit jam), milk

- ◆ ½ bagel, 1 teaspoon peanut butter, 1 teaspoon jam, 1 cup fat-free milk
- ■ 1 bagel, 2 teaspoons peanut butter, 2 teaspoons jam, 1 cup fat-free milk
- ● ½ bagel, ½ to 1 teaspoon peanut butter, ½ to 1 teaspoon jam, ½ to 1 cup low-fat milk

SNACK

Fresh Homemade Salsa (page 260) with baked chips

- ◆ Salsa, 6 chips
- ■ Salsa, 12 chips
- ● Salsa, 4 to 6 chips

Zesty Tuna Salad (page 242) on whole grain crackers, dried apricots

- ◆ ¼ serving tuna, 3 crackers, 3 apricots
- ■ ½ serving tuna, 6 crackers, 4 apricots
- ● ¼ serving tuna, 2 or 3 crackers, 1 or 2 apricots

Low-fat cottage cheese and fresh cherries

- ◆ ¼ cup cottage cheese, 6 cherries
- ■ ½ cup cottage cheese, 12 cherries
- ● 2 to 4 tablespoons cottage cheese, 4 to 6 cherries

DINNER

Lean roast pork tenderloin; whole wheat pasta sprinkled with Parmesan cheese; Broccoli, Orange, and Watercress Salad (page 257)

- ◆ 3 ounces pork, ½ cup pasta, 1 serving salad
- ■ 4 ounces pork, 1 cup pasta, 1 serving salad
- ● 1 to 2 ounces pork, ¼ to ½ cup pasta, ¼ to ½ serving salad

Homemade Pita Pizzas (page 245), side salad with olive oil vinaigrette, milk

- ◆ 1 pizza, 1 cup salad with 1 teaspoon olive oil and balsamic vinegar, 1 cup fat-free milk
- ■ 2 pizzas, 1 cup salad with 1 teaspoon olive oil and balsamic vinegar, 1 cup fat-free milk
- ● ½ to 1 pizza, ¼ to ½ cup salad with ½ teaspoon olive oil and balsamic vinegar, ½ to 1 cup low-fat milk

Chicken or tofu stir-fry with broccoli, water chestnuts, and carrots; brown rice; milk

- ◆ 3 ounces chicken or tofu with vegetables, ⅓ cup rice, 1 cup fat-free milk

- 4 ounces chicken or tofu with vegetables, ⅔ cup rice, 1 cup fat-free milk

- 2 to 3 ounces chicken or tofu with vegetables, 2 to 4 tablespoons rice, ½ to 1 cup low-fat milk

▼SATURDAY

Choose one option for each meal and snack.

BREAKFAST

Whole Wheat Pancakes (page 239), low-fat or vegetarian sausage

- ◆ 2 pancakes, 2 pieces sausage

- ■ 3 pancakes, 3 pieces sausage

- ● 1 or 2 pancakes, 1 or 2 pieces sausage

Spinach and Feta Omelet (page 238)

- ◆ 1 serving omelet

- ■ 1 serving omelet

- ● ¼ to ½ serving omelet

Oatmeal with milk

- ◆ ½ cup oatmeal, 1 tablespoon protein powder, 1 cup fat-free milk

- ■ 1 cup oatmeal, 2 tablespoons protein powder, 1 cup fat-free milk

- ● ½ to 1 cup oatmeal, ½ to 1 cup low-fat milk

SNACK

Spinach and Artichoke Heart Dip (page 261) with small baked whole wheat pita

- ◆ 1 serving dip, 1 pita

- ■ 1½ servings dip, 1 pita

- ● ½ to 1 serving dip, ½ to 1 pita

One-half peanut butter and banana sandwich (with all-natural peanut butter)

- ◆ ½ slice bread, ½ teaspoon peanut butter, ¼ banana

- ■ ½ slice bread, 1 teaspoon peanut butter, ¼ banana

- ● ¼ to ½ slice bread, ½ teaspoon peanut butter, ¼ banana

Popcorn, turkey slices with fresh tomatoes sprinkled with lemon pepper

- ◆ 3 cups popcorn, 1 ounce turkey, tomatoes

- ■ 3 cups popcorn, 2 ounces turkey, tomatoes

- ● 1 cup popcorn, ½ ounce turkey, tomatoes

LUNCH (EAT IN)

Sweet Potato Minestrone (page 246), grilled chicken

- ◆ 1 serving soup, 2 ounces chicken

- ■ 1 serving soup, 3 ounces chicken

- ● ½ serving soup, 1 to 2 ounces chicken

Zesty Tuna Salad (page 242) over whole wheat angel hair pasta, steamed carrots, milk

- ◆ ½ serving tuna, ½ cup pasta, carrots, 1 cup fat-free milk

- ■ ½ serving tuna, 1 cup pasta, carrots, 1 cup fat-free milk

- ● ¼ to ½ serving tuna, ¼ cup pasta, carrots, ½ to 1 cup low-fat milk

LUNCH (EAT OUT)

Spaghetti marinara, side salad with olive oil vinaigrette

- ◆ ½ cup spaghetti, 1 meatball, 1 cup salad with 1 teaspoon olive oil and balsamic vinegar

- ■ 1 cup spaghetti, 1 meatball, 1 cup salad with 1 teaspoon olive oil and balsamic vinegar

- ● ¼ to ½ cup spaghetti, ½ to 1 meatball, ¼ to ½ cup salad with ½ to 1 teaspoon olive oil and balsamic vinegar

SNACK

White bean dip with carrots and small whole wheat pita

- ◆ ¼ cup dip, carrots, ½ pita

- ■ ¼ cup dip, carrots, 1 pita

- ● 2 tablespoons dip, carrots, ½ pita

Celery with thinly spread peanut butter topped with raisins

- ◆ 1 rib celery, 1 teaspoon peanut butter, 1 tablespoon raisins

- ■ 1 rib celery, 1 teaspoon peanut butter, 1 tablespoon raisins, 1 ounce turkey

- ● ½ to 1 rib celery, ½ to 1 teaspoon peanut butter, ½ to 1 tablespoon raisins

Veggie Dip (page 262) with fresh-cut vegetables

- ◆ 1 serving dip, vegetables

- ■ 2 servings dip, vegetables

- ● ½ serving dip, vegetables

DINNER

Baked Fish with Vegetables (page 250), whole wheat rotini with freshly grated Parmesan cheese

- ◆ 1 serving fish with vegetables, ½ cup rotini, 1 ounce cheese

- ■ 1 serving fish with vegetables, 1 cup rotini, 1 ounce cheese

- ● ½ serving fish with vegetables, ¼ cup rotini, ½ to 1 ounce cheese

Soft tacos made with whole wheat tortillas, grilled steak or chicken, tomatoes, lettuce, grilled peppers, and low-fat cheese; milk

- ◆ 2 tortillas, 3 ounces meat, tomatoes, lettuce, and peppers, 1 ounce cheese, 1 cup fat-free milk

- ■ 3 tortillas, 4 ounces meat, tomatoes, lettuce, and peppers, 1 ounce cheese, 1 cup fat-free milk

- ● 1 tortilla, 1 to 2 ounces meat, tomatoes, lettuce, and peppers, ½ to 1 ounce cheese, ½ to 1 cup low-fat milk

Sloppy Joes (page 252) on whole grain bun, Baked French Fries (page 255), side salad with olive oil vinaigrette, milk

- ◆ 1 bun, 1 serving Sloppy Joes, ½ serving fries, 1 cup salad with 1 teaspoon olive oil and balsamic vinegar, 1 cup fat-free milk

- ■ 1 bun, 1 serving Sloppy Joes, 1 serving fries, 1 cup salad with 1 teaspoon olive oil and balsamic vinegar, 1 cup fat-free milk

- ● ½ bun, ¼ to ½ serving Sloppy Joes, ¼ to ½ serving fries, ¼ to ½ cup salad with ½ teaspoon olive oil and balsamic vinegar, ½ to 1 cup low-fat milk

▼ SUNDAY

Choose one option for each meal and snack.

BREAKFAST

Shrimp and Veggie Omelet (page 240) with whole grain toast

- ◆ 1 serving omelet, 1 slice toast

- ■ 1 serving omelet, 1 slice toast

- ● ¼ to ½ serving omelet, ½ to 1 slice toast

French toast made with whole grain bread, low-fat or vegetarian sausage

- ◆ 2 slices French toast, 1 piece sausage

- ■ 3 slices French toast, 2 pieces sausage

- ● ½ to 1 slice French toast, 1 piece sausage

Low-fat vanilla yogurt with orange slices

- ◆ ½ cup yogurt mixed with ¼ cup cottage cheese, ½ orange

- ■ 1 cup yogurt mixed with ¼ cup cottage cheese, ½ orange

- ● ¼ to ½ cup yogurt, ¼ orange

SNACK

Low-fat cottage cheese mixed with low-fat sour cream and sprinkled with brown sugar and cinnamon, with fresh fruit for dipping

- ◆ ¼ cup cottage cheese, 1 tablespoon sour cream, ½ cup fruit

- ■ ½ cup cottage cheese, 1 tablespoon sour cream, ½ cup fruit

- ● 2 to 3 tablespoons cottage cheese, ½ tablespoon sour cream, ¼ cup fruit

Apple Ladybug Treats (page 260)

- ◆ 1 serving treats, 1 ounce turkey

- ■ 1 serving treats, 2 ounces turkey

- ● 1 serving treats

Reduced-fat mozzarella sticks and grapes

- ◆ 1 cheese stick, 15 grapes

- ■ 2 cheese sticks, 15 grapes

- ● ½ cheese stick, 6 to 10 grapes

LUNCH (EAT IN)

Chicken Salad (page 244), whole grain bread, apple slices

- ◆ 1 slice bread, 1 serving chicken salad, 1 apple

- ■ 1 slice bread, 1 serving chicken salad, 1 apple

- ● ½ to 1 slice bread, ¼ to ½ serving chicken salad, ¼ to ½ apple

Roast beef sandwich on whole grain bread, side salad with olive oil vinaigrette, cantaloupe cubes

- ◆ 1 slice bread, 2 ounces roast beef, 1 cup salad with 1 teaspoon olive oil and balsamic vinegar, 1 cup cantaloupe cubes

- ■ 2 slices bread, 3 ounces roast beef, 1 cup salad with 1 teaspoon olive oil and balsamic vinegar, 1 cup cantaloupe cubes

- ● 1 slice bread, 1 to 2 ounces roast beef, ½ cup salad with ½ teaspoon olive oil and balsamic vinegar, ¼ to ½ cup cantaloupe cubes

LUNCH (EAT OUT)

Chicken and vegetable stir-fry with brown rice, milk

- ◆ 2 ounces chicken with vegetables, ⅓ cup rice, 1 cup fat-free milk

- ■ 3 ounces chicken with vegetables, ⅔ cup rice, 1 cup fat-free milk

- ● 1 to 2 ounces chicken with vegetables, 2 to 4 tablespoons rice, ½ to 1 cup low-fat milk

SNACK

Protein bar (14+ grams protein, 25 grams carbohydrates, less than 3 grams fat)

- ◆ ½ energy bar

- ■ 1 energy bar

- ● ¼ to ½ energy bar

Fruit Smoothie (page 263)

- ◆ ½ serving smoothie

- ■ 1 serving smoothie, 2 tablespoons protein powder

- ● ¼ serving smoothie

Trail mix made with Wheat Chex, raisins, and peanuts or almonds

- ◆ ¼ cup Wheat Chex, 1 tablespoon raisins, ½ tablespoon nuts

- ■ ½ cup Wheat Chex, 2 tablespoons raisins, 1 tablespoon nuts

- ● ¼ to ½ cup Wheat Chex, ½ to 1 tablespoon raisins, ½ tablespoon nuts

DINNER

Cajun-Spiced Chicken (page 247), brown rice, steamed green beans, milk

- ◆ 1 serving chicken, ⅓ cup rice, green beans, 1 cup fat-free milk

- ■ 1 serving chicken, ⅔ cup rice, green beans, 1 cup fat-free milk

- ● ¼ to ½ serving chicken, 2 to 4 tablespoons rice, green beans, ½ to 1 cup low-fat milk

Cabbage Roll-Ups (page 249), side salad with olive oil vinaigrette

- ◆ 1 serving roll-ups, 1 cup salad with 1 teaspoon olive oil and balsamic vinegar

- ■ 1½ servings roll-ups, 1 cup salad with 1 teaspoon olive oil and balsamic vinegar

- ● ¼ to ½ serving roll-ups, ¼ to ½ cup salad with ½ teaspoon olive oil and balsamic vinegar

Grilled lean steak, Roasted Vegetables (page 259), red potatoes

- ◆ 3 ounces steak, 1 serving vegetables, 1 cup potatoes

- ■ 4 ounces steak, 1 serving vegetables, 1½ cups potatoes

- ● 2 to 3 ounces steak, ½ to 1 serving vegetables, ½ to 1 cup potatoes

FITNESS FOCUS

This is going to be fun! In Week 5, as promised, I'm going to share some of my very own exercise routines that I use with my clients every day. I use these workouts to keep my clients focused, motivated, and successful in reaching their goals. The exercise routines in this chapter feature interval-training techniques that are wonderfully effective. Now that you have mastered the basics during the first 4 weeks, these routines will help you put it all together to create more weight loss and muscle toning. I am excited and honored to share them with you.

SENA SAYS:
Big results tomorrow come from doing the little things today. Be successful—take action.

One quick thing before we move on: I want to make sure everyone is writing down their activities for the week. Did your son ride his bike and take those foul shots as he said he would? Did your daughter get her cardio in and stretch a little, so that she's happy, having fun, and ready for next year's cheerleading squad? That reminder is for you too, Mom.

Week 5: Interval Routines

Okay, it's time to reveal one of the key reasons that my clients are so often delighted with the slimming-down, firming-up results of their programs. It's called interval training, and though it sounds as if it might be difficult or complicated, it's really quite simple.

With interval training, you go through your routine of strength-training exercises as I've shown you. But now, between every two or three exercises, you add an interval of brisk cardio work. So easy, but so effective!

Interval training really kicks the fat-burning process into high gear. There's nothing else like it. When my clients get going for a week or two with this new addition to their routines, they really see the pounds melt off.

SENA SAYS:
You win—fat loses. That's the way I expect this "game" to end!

Intervals are both challenging and effective. Always use your best judgment regarding your exertion levels. Be careful not to exceed your R.P.E. level (beginners 4 to 6, intermediate 6 to 8, and advanced 8 to 10). Be sure that you always feel safe and comfortable when you are exercising. Stop immediately if you feel faint, dizzy, or lightheaded.

Now let's put our interval routines into action.

For Adults (Age 18 and Older)

Refer back to the strength-training exercise circuit that I recommended in Week 2. I want to have you work within that same template, adding three intervals of cardiovascular activity.

With each interval of cardio, you will increase the time by 15 seconds. Thus, if your first interval was 30 seconds long, your second will be 45 seconds and the third 60 seconds. It's simple. You just perform a couple of strength-training exercises and then a different activity that challenges the body with change.

Cardiovascular exercises for intervals can include High Steps (page 207), High Marches (page 209), climbing stairs, walking on a treadmill, or doing what I call sports-specific movements.

Sports-specific movements are like practicing sports—without the game. Try mimicking swinging a bat, throwing a ball, or shadow boxing. If you play basketball, pretend to shoot or dribble. You don't need the actual equipment; just repeat the mechanics of the particular sports movement. Today's professional athletes are using the same techniques and methods to condition their bodies to perform at high levels.

You can also try . . .

❏ Golf swings   ❏ Football tosses

❏ Soccer kicks   ❏ Martial arts kicks

My recommended personal training routine for adults follows. If you are ready to turn it up a notch, try starting with longer intervals and continue to increase them by 15 seconds each time.

❏ In between exercises #2 and #3, do an interval of a cardiovascular movement for 30 seconds.

❏ In between exercises #5 and #6, perform an interval of a sports-specific movement for 45 seconds, repeating it for improved form and for conditioning.

❏ After exercise #8, do another interval of cardiovascular activity for 60 seconds.

Overall, your strength-training and interval routine will look like this:

#1: Chest Presses

#2: Back Rows

Interval—Cardiovascular activity (30 seconds to 2 minutes)

#3: Triceps Pushdowns

#4: Abdominal Crunches

#5: Biceps Curls

Interval—Sports-specific movements (30 seconds to 2 minutes)

#6: Shoulder Presses

#7: Back Extensions

#8: Leg Squats

Interval—Cardiovascular movement (30 seconds to 2 minutes)

(Add 15 seconds each interval)

If you are doing more than one strength-training circuit at a time, try doing two intervals of sports-specific movements and one of cardiovascular activity during this second go-round. Keep changing and mixing it up whenever you can. This is an effective tool for athletes around the world—and now you can benefit from it as well!

Interval training is part of your strength-training program: All cardiovascular exercise, core movements, and flexibility stretches are separate and should always be completed.

For Teenagers (Ages 13 to 17)

Teenage boys and girls should use the strength-training routine that I recommended in Week 2. They just need to add an interval of a cardiovascular activity or a sports-specific movement, such as a batting swing, golf swing, or basketball shot. Within this interval, regardless of what teens choose, their cardiovascular activity should last from 30 seconds to 2 minutes (if they're advanced).

In between exercises #2 and #3, have your teen perform the following exercise.

HIGH STEP

(ABDOMEN, BACK, HIPS, LEGS)

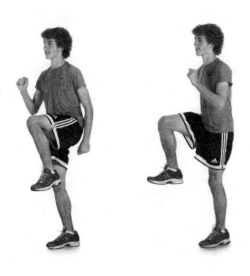

Here's how: Start with your feet shoulder width apart, knees soft, abdomen firm, and elbows bent at 90 degrees. Slowly start to pump your legs, lifting first one leg and then the other. Progress toward rapid speed as you pump your legs, and move your arms as well. Breathe continuously and keep your eyes open. You can look down at the floor if it improves your balance.

In between exercises #5 and #6, have your teen perform a sports-specific movement. Overall, teens' routines will look like this:

#1: Chest Presses (with tubes)

#2: Back Rows (with tubes)

Interval—High Steps (30 seconds to 2 minutes)

#3: Triceps Pushdowns

#4: Abdominal Crunches

#5: Biceps Curls

Interval—Sports-specific movements (30 seconds to 2 minutes)

#6: Shoulder Presses

#7: Back Extensions

#8: Leg Squats

For Children (Age 12 and Younger)

Keep it simple, but accelerate your kids' program and results. Try this anytime you would like to have your child do something a little different and add some challenge to their activities.

In between exercises #2 and #3, have your child perform the following exercise.

HIGH MARCH

(ABDOMEN, BACK, HIPS, LEGS)

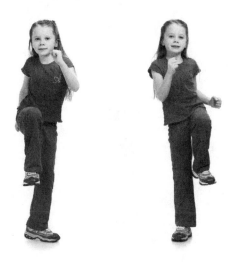

Here's how: Stand with your feet shoulder width apart, knees soft, abdomen firm, and elbows bent at 90 degrees. First, slowly lift one knee as high as you can without losing your balance, then return to the starting position. Repeat with the other leg, then continue to lift one leg after the other. Keep your eyes open and your head and neck neutral, and breathe normally. Do 10 repetitions per leg, catch your breath, then move on to exercise #3.

Next, in between exercises #5 and #6, have your child do the following exercise.

ONE-LEG HOP

(ANKLES, CALVES, LEGS, HIPS)

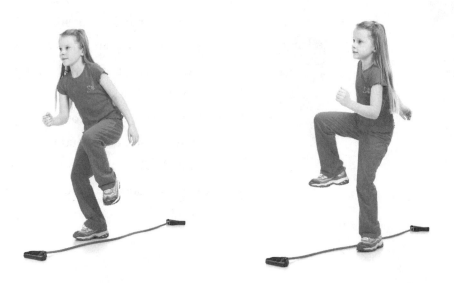

Here's how: Start by standing with your feet together on one side of a tube or rope, knees soft, abdomen firm, head and neck neutral, and eyes open. Lift your right leg off the floor and try to hop to the other side of the tube or rope using your other leg. Try 5 hops on the left leg, then 5 hops on the right, and then repeat with 5 more on each leg. Catch your breath, then move on to exercise #6.

(If your child is unable to perform this exercise safely or experiences knee pain, have her stop immediately. Instead, have her repeat High March.)

Overall, your child's strength-training and interval routine will look like this:

#1: Pushups

#2: Back Extensions

Interval—High March: 10 reps

#3: Biceps Curls

#4: Overhead Presses

#5: Sit/Stand Chair Exercises

Interval—One-Leg Hop or High March: 10 reps per leg

#6: Abdominal Crunches

#7: One-Leg Balances

FIT FAMILY ACTIVITY

Let's shoot some hoops. Of course, what I mean is play basketball, one of the world's most beloved sports, which is played in hundreds of countries and growing more popular all the time.

Since it's so popular, you may already have a basketball rim and net right in your yard or at a nearby park. That's great! But when was the last time you picked up a ball and used the court, or better yet, played basketball as a family? Get going to the basement or garage and get that basketball out, put some air in it, and gather up your family for some healthy fun!

I have been playing basketball since I was 7, and I still love to play today. It has been my favorite sport throughout all these years. Here are some ideas for you and your family to have a ball. (Remember to have ice and a first-aid kit close by, just in case.)

Not everyone in your family may be able to play an actual game. If they can, great! If not, try something else, such as shooting contests. My favorite is a foul-shooting contest. Have each family member take three shots in a row and then rotate shooters, and have someone keep score. How about a game of "Horse"? This is where one family member goes first by being creative with a shot—any kind of shot from anywhere on the court. She could shoot overhand, underhand, do a hook shot, or take a layup with her eyes closed. If she makes the shot, then everyone else in the family has to take an identical shot. If you don't make it, you get the letter H. Then someone else makes up a shot, and those who don't make it get a letter O. Whoever spells out "horse" first is out of the game. Take some crazy shots and have a blast!

You could also see who can dribble the longest, between their legs, or behind their backs. Or how about "Who can spin the ball on their fingertips?" I know how much fun basketball can be—share it with your family and get healthy at the same time!

One of the wonderful things about basketball is that it is a great sport outside on a neighborhood court or inside if the weather isn't great. Lots of local schools have open time on the weekends at their gymnasium courts. You can also play at the Y, the community center, or a park district gym. (For other activities, see appendix B.)

WEEK 5 FINAL THOUGHTS

As a personal trainer, I am asked the same question over and over again: "How do I get results fast?" My answer is always the same: "Turn up the volume." Put an extra 10 to 20 percent more effort into your exercise sessions and eat really well, with no deviating from your meal plans.

Pick up the intensity of your focus, and you will witness more results. I'm telling you "the facts, ma'am, just the facts." I'll see you and the gang in our sixth and final week!

WEEK 5 ACTION STEP SUMMARY

❑ Hold your Week 5 Fit Family Meeting.

❑ Make adjustments to your strategies where needed.

❑ Review food diaries—be on the lookout for unhealthy fats and sugar.

❑ Review exercise/activity journals—are family members keeping exercise commitments?

❑ Focus on healthy snacks and desserts.

❑ Add intervals to your exercise routine.

❑ Play a family basketball game—outside or inside.

❑ Schedule your Week 6 Fit Family Meeting.

WEEK 6

Lean Mom and Beyond

Today's meeting will mark the start of a very important week. This is not only the grand finale of our 6-week program, it is also the time when everyone should be zeroing in on their individual goals. It's the final week where, as a family and as individuals, you can focus on your goals and strategies and make sure that they are perfectly aligned for success in the future.

JUST FOR YOU, MOM

I must admit, this is an exciting moment for me. I get to pass the torch to you fully, so that you can become the coach of your family's health and fitness lifestyles! No one is better suited or equipped to guide your family toward a life of feeling good, being healthy, and having increased confidence and improved self-esteem. No one can better prepare your family to avoid unhealthy foods, have some fun through regular activity, and, at the same time, stave off a lifetime of unnecessary illness.

You now know how to do this for your family and for yourself. Always remember, whether it's Week 6, Week 16, Week 46, or 6 years from now, when you follow my recommendations, you will get results. Just take it 1 week at a time.

You will lose weight this week, Mom, if you:

❏ Try two full strength-training circuit routines with intervals (burns calories from fat more efficiently and increases metabolism and toning).

❏ Change your cardiovascular activity again (avoids plateaus and boredom).

❏ Refrain from having any fancy coffee drinks or sodas this week (cuts calorie and sugar intake).

❏ Try to finish dinner more than 4 hours prior to bedtime (boosts weight loss—big time). Eating close to bedtime doesn't give you much chance to burn off calories, so you're more likely put on weight. If you work late and just can't eat early, try to make dinner a light meal or try to get some exercise before bedtime with a walk around the block or some crunches.

WEEK 6 FIT FAMILY MEETING AGENDA

❏ Review individual goals—did your family members meet them?

❏ Review food diaries and exercise/activity journals—did you adopt each principle of weight management from chapter 1?

❏ Discuss your meal planning and Week 6 Food Focus: dining out.

❏ Discuss and plan your Week 6 Fitness Focus: Design your own personal routine.

❏ Fit Family Activity: An outing to celebrate goals achieved and a new healthy lifestyle.

WEEK 6 FIT FAMILY MEETING

Way back when we started, we discussed short-term goals, long-term goals, and the strategies to achieve them. Everyone in your family wrote them down, right? Your Week 6 Fit Family Meeting is the perfect time to pull out your goal sheets and see what each person has actually accomplished. Turn back to page 36 and have every family member take the Fit Family Quiz one more time. Look at your changed scores, then go around the room and discuss how everyone has done. We don't need to be judgmental, but we do need to be honest. If you stayed with my plan, you probably reached most—if not all—of your goals. I also understand that this is real life, and you or other family members may have wavered from the plan from time to time. You may not have achieved all of the success that you envisioned. If that's the case, don't give up! Just remember to make better choices next time.

The important thing now is that you determine what is working and what isn't. Then develop strategies to correct the things that aren't going as planned—adjustments are a key to success!

At the beginning of our program, we asked each family member to make a commitment to the rest of the group. Has everyone done what they committed to do, and has each family member been a support to the family

SENA SAYS:

If you haven't reached all of your goals, don't fret. Remember, this is a 6-week plan, and fitness is a way of life. You have plenty of time to perfect your program!

as a group? These are important questions that you want to address now, before Week 6 starts. You and your family will need these tools beyond this 6-week program so you can continue to be successful. Never underestimate the importance of these commitments; make any needed adjustments now.

Remember, I designed my 6-week plan around the involvement of the entire family. When each person is pulling his or her respective load, it's amazing how successful the family plan becomes. One of the nice side benefits of this program is that your family has done this together. Many families have told me that the togetherness that they achieved through this common mission was just as rewarding as the weight-loss and fitness results.

Now that you've looked at each family member's goals and commitment, let's go to it!

REVIEW YOUR FOOD DIARIES

Wow! Your family has made it to the last week! As everyone reviews their food diaries, look back from Week 1 on to assess all of the positive changes they have made. Take the time to compliment your family on the hard work they've done. Although you may not have reached all of your goals, your list of changes can serve as a constant reminder of what you are capable of achieving when you try. It will be a motivator as you continue on your journey to reach your nutritional goals.

Let's review the focus points of the past 5 weeks. Ask yourself how you have done in each of these areas.

❑ Keeping a daily record of your food intake in your food diaries

❑ Drinking 8 to 10 cups of water a day

❑ Monitoring portion sizes and paying attention to your level of fullness so you don't overeat

❑ Decreasing sugary drinks to one or none per day

❑ Eating lean protein and fiber with each meal and snack

❑ Replacing simple carbohydrates with complex carbohydrates (such as replacing white rice with brown rice)

❑ Eating small meals and snacks at least every 3 hours during the day

❑ Increasing the amount of fruits and vegetables to an ultimate goal of five or more servings a day

❑ Decreasing the amount of unhealthy fats to one serving per day and concentrating on using healthy fats for the fat servings in your meal plan

❑ Decreasing the amount of processed foods and fast foods in your meal plans

Over the past 6 weeks, I have given your family a great deal of nutrition information on which to concentrate. If some of these changes have felt overwhelming, or if your family has had difficulty keeping them up, go back to the first week and go through the program again, 1 week at a time.

Maybe you have been stressed or distracted or so busy that you just couldn't focus. Or perhaps certain family members just weren't ready to change. Either way, don't worry. Just go back to Week 1 and try again. We're going for a lifetime behavior change, so another 6 weeks is no big deal. Simply go back and work on each week until you feel you have mastered the exercises and nutrition advice. Just remember to consistently continue to work on the changes that will help your family reach their goals—and always remind each other that you *can* do it! Now, let's get going on our Week 6 Food Focus.

WEEK 6 FOOD FOCUS: DINING OUT

Back in Week 2, my food focus was on lunches, and I discussed different fast-food restaurants and the healthy choices they offer. Although fast food is a popular choice for a quick lunch, many of us also enjoy going out for a more relaxing meal. My focus this week is on making healthier choices when eating out in a more traditional restaurant setting or when ordering food in. I will include some recommendations for specific ethnic cuisine as well as general rules to follow when looking at a menu.

I really enjoy eating out and do so several times a week. However, I don't always choose items directly from the menu. Instead, I often look at the types of food the restaurant offers and make special requests if I don't see something that fits into my meal plan. For example, most restaurants have fish, chicken breasts, or a lean cut of beef or pork that they can prepare without added fat. I add a side of vegetables or a salad (with olive oil and vinegar dressing) with brown rice or a baked potato without butter or sour cream. I end up with a great, healthy meal that fits my meal plan and allows me to enjoy dining out.

I'm a big fan of stir-fry restaurants where you pick all the "fixings," and the chef does the cooking. There is always a great selection of lean protein choices, fresh vegetables, and brown rice—and best of all, you have complete control over what is being added to your meal. Here are some general tips for ordering food.

- ❏ Don't be afraid to make a special request or to order à la carte if you don't see a healthy option on the menu.
- ❏ Split an entrée with a friend or your spouse and order a salad on the side.
- ❏ Order appetizer-size portions or take half of the food home.
- ❏ Monitor alcohol intake and avoid high-sugar, frozen mixed drinks such as margaritas and piña coladas.

Some terms and phrases that indicate low-fat preparation are *steamed, poached, lemon, charbroiled, roasted, marinara, boiled, in tomato sauce, in its own juice,* and *baked.*

Terms and phrases that warn of high-fat preparation include *buttery, fried, in butter sauce, sautéed, fried, pan-fried, scalloped, braised, creamed, in cream sauce, hollandaise, crispy, au gratin, in cheese sauce, battered, prime, hash,* and *au fromage.*

Here are guidelines for various ethnic cuisines, whether you're eating out or ordering in.

Mexican

❏ Avoid foods that are fried.

❏ Eat soft tortillas as opposed to chips or taco shells. Limit the number you eat.

❏ Ask to have cheese, sour cream, and guacamole left off the top of your dish and limited in the ingredients.

❏ Guacamole is a very high-fat choice, while salsa is fat-free (although avocados contain a "good" fat, a portion is only ⅛ of an avocado).

Italian

❏ Choose red sauces instead of alfredo or cheese sauce.

❏ Ask for an appetizer-size portion of your pasta dish or split it with someone.

❏ Fill one-third to one-half of your plate with salad.

❏ Limit bread before and with the meal, and be aware that garlic bread is usually loaded with butter.

Chinese

❏ Avoid items that are fried, such as egg rolls and sweet and sour chicken.

❏ Choose items with lots of vegetables and unbreaded meat or seafood.

❏ Select steamed rice instead of fried rice.

Thai

❏ Choose broth-based soups with lots of vegetables and lean meat or seafood as an entrée.

❏ Unfried spring rolls are a great choice.

❏ Watch your portions with noodle dishes or share with a friend or family member.

Pizza

❏ Choose thin crust instead of thick or stuffed crust.

❏ Ask for a smaller amount of cheese to be added.

❏ Load up the pizza with vegetables.

❏ Choose lean meats such as chicken breast and lean sirloin as toppings.

WEEK 6 MEAL PLANS

◆ = goal weight 160 pounds or lower

■ = goal weight over 160 pounds

● = kids age 12 and under

▼ MONDAY

Choose one option for each meal and snack.

BREAKFAST

High-fiber, high-protein cereal with milk

◆ ½ cup cereal, 3 tablespoons protein powder, 1 cup fat-free milk

■ 1 cup cereal, 3 tablespoons protein powder, 1 cup fat-free milk

● ½ to 1 cup cereal, ½ to 1 cup low-fat milk

Low-fat vanilla yogurt with fresh blueberries

◆ 1 cup yogurt, ¾ cup blueberries

■ 1½ cups yogurt, ¾ cup blueberries

● ½ to 1 cup yogurt, ¼ to ½ cup blueberries

Whole grain waffles, low-fat or vegetarian sausage

◆ 2 waffles, 2 pieces sausage

■ 3 waffles, 3 pieces sausage

● 1 to 1½ waffles, 1 piece sausage

SNACK

Soy nuts and dried apricots

◆ ¼ cup soy nuts, 2 apricots

■ ¼ cup soy nuts, 2 apricots

● 2 to 3 tablespoons soy nuts, 1 apricot

Celery with thinly spread peanut butter topped with raisins

◆ 1 rib celery, 1 teaspoon peanut butter, 1 tablespoon raisins

- 1 rib celery, 1 teaspoon peanut butter, 1 tablespoon raisins, 1 ounce turkey

- ½ to 1 rib celery, ½ to 1 teaspoon peanut butter, ½ to 1 tablespoon raisins

Whole wheat graham crackers dipped in low-fat vanilla yogurt

- 1 cracker, 4 tablespoons yogurt

- 1 cracker, 4 tablespoons yogurt

- ½ to 1 cracker, 2 to 4 tablespoons yogurt

LUNCH (EAT IN)

Couscous with Portobello Mushrooms and Sun-Dried Tomatoes (page 241), grilled chicken, grapes

- 1 serving couscous, 2 ounces chicken, 7 grapes

- 1 serving couscous, 3 ounces chicken, 15 grapes

- ¼ to ½ serving couscous, 1 to 2 ounces chicken, 4 to 6 grapes

LUNCH (EAT OUT)

Subway honey mustard ham wrap

- 1 wrap

- 1 wrap

- ¼ to ½ wrap

LUNCH (AT SCHOOL)

Egg Salad (page 242) on whole grain roll, grapes, baby carrots

- 1 small roll, 1 serving egg salad, 15 grapes, carrots

- 1 medium roll, 1 serving egg salad, 15 grapes, carrots

- ½ to 1 small roll, ¼ to ½ serving egg salad, 6 to 10 grapes, carrots

SNACK

Trail mix made with Wheat Chex, raisins, and peanuts or almonds

- ¼ cup Wheat Chex, 1 tablespoon raisins, ½ tablespoon nuts

- ½ cup Wheat Chex, 2 tablespoons raisins, 1 tablespoon nuts

- ¼ to ½ cup Wheat Chex, ½ to 1 tablespoon raisins, ½ tablespoon nuts

Low-fat vanilla yogurt with fresh strawberries

- ½ cup yogurt, ¼ cup strawberries

- ¾ cup yogurt, ½ cup strawberries

- ¼ to ½ cup yogurt, ¼ cup strawberries

Edamame (soybeans)—buy fresh or frozen and boil. If precooked, heat in microwave.

- ½ cup edamame

- 1 cup edamame

- ¼ cup edamame

DINNER

Homemade Pita Pizzas (page 245), side salad with olive oil vinaigrette, milk

- 1 pizza, 1 cup salad with 1 teaspoon olive oil and balsamic vinegar, 1 cup fat-free milk

- ■ 2 pizzas, 1 cup salad with 1 teaspoon olive oil and balsamic vinegar, 1 cup fat-free milk

- ● ½ to 1 pizza, ¼ to ½ cup salad with ½ teaspoon olive oil and balsamic vinegar, ½ to 1 cup low-fat milk

Sloppy Joes (page 252) on whole grain bun, side salad with olive oil vinaigrette, milk

- ◆ 1 bun, 1 serving Sloppy Joes, 1 cup salad with 1 teaspoon olive oil and balsamic vinegar, 1 cup fat-free milk

- ■ 1 bun, 1 serving Sloppy Joes, 1 cup salad with 1 teaspoon olive oil and balsamic vinegar, 1 cup fat-free milk

- ● ½ bun, ¼ to ½ serving Sloppy Joes, ½ to 1 cup salad with ½ teaspoon olive oil and balsamic vinegar, ½ to 1 cup low-fat milk

Grilled Salmon (page 245), baked potato with low-fat sour cream, steamed carrots, milk

- ◆ 1 serving salmon, 1 small potato with 2 tablespoons sour cream, carrots, 1 cup fat-free milk

- ■ 1 serving salmon, 1 medium potato with 2 tablespoons sour cream, carrots, 1 cup fat-free milk

- ● ½ serving salmon, ½ small potato with 1 tablespoon sour cream, carrots, ½ to 1 cup low-fat milk

▼TUESDAY

Choose one option for each meal and snack.

BREAKFAST

Oatmeal with milk

- ◆ ½ cup oatmeal, 1 tablespoon protein powder, 1 cup fat-free milk

- ■ 1 cup oatmeal, 2 tablespoons protein powder, 1 cup fat-free milk

- ● ½ to 1 cup oatmeal, ½ to 1 cup low-fat milk

Low-fat cheese melted on whole grain toast

- ◆ 2 ounces cheese, 2 slices toast

- ■ 2 ounces cheese, 2 slices toast, 1 cup fat-free milk

- ● 1 ounce cheese, ½ to 1 slice toast

Spinach and Feta Omelet (page 238)

- ◆ 1 serving omelet

- ■ 1 serving omelet

- ● ¼ to ½ serving omelet

SNACK

Low-fat vanilla yogurt mixed with fresh strawberries and sprinkled with sunflower seeds

- ◆ ½ cup yogurt, ½ cup strawberries, 1 tablespoon sunflower seeds

- ■ ½ cup yogurt, ½ cup strawberries, 1 tablespoon sunflower seeds

- ● ¼ to ½ cup yogurt, ¼ to ½ cup strawberries, 1 teaspoon sunflower seeds

One-half turkey sandwich with tomato slices sprinkled with lemon pepper

- ◆ 1 slice bread, 1 ounce turkey, tomatoes
- ■ 1 slice bread, 2 ounces turkey, tomatoes
- ● ½ slice bread, ½ ounce turkey, tomatoes

Hard-cooked egg on whole grain toast

- ◆ 1 egg, 1 slice toast
- ■ 1 egg and 1 egg white, 1 slice toast
- ● ½ egg, ½ slice toast

LUNCH (EAT IN)

Sweet Potato Minestrone (page 246), grilled chicken

- ◆ 1 serving soup, 2 ounces chicken
- ■ 1 serving soup, 3 ounces chicken
- ● ½ serving soup, 1 to 2 ounces chicken

LUNCH (EAT OUT)

Boston Market rotisserie chicken, butternut squash, sesame broccoli

- ◆ 2 ounces chicken, ½ cup squash, 1 cup broccoli
- ■ 3 ounces chicken, 1 cup squash, 1 cup broccoli
- ● 1 to 2 ounces chicken, ¼ cup squash, ¼ to ½ cup broccoli

LUNCH (AT SCHOOL)

Turkey, lettuce, and tomato on whole wheat tortilla, cantaloupe cubes

- ◆ 1 tortilla, 2 ounces turkey, lettuce, tomato slices, 1 cup cantaloupe cubes

- ■ 2 tortillas, 3 ounces turkey, lettuce, tomato slices, 1 cup cantaloupe cubes
- ● ½ tortilla, 1 to 2 ounces turkey, lettuce, tomato slices, ¼ to ½ cup cantaloupe cubes

SNACK

Fresh Homemade Salsa (page 260) with baked chips

- ◆ Salsa, 6 chips
- ■ Salsa, 12 chips
- ● Salsa, 6 chips

Small toasted whole wheat pita with fat-free refried beans

- ◆ 1 pita, ¼ cup beans
- ■ 1 pita, ¼ cup beans
- ● ½ pita, 2 tablespoons beans

Celery with thinly spread peanut butter topped with raisins

- ◆ 1 rib celery, 1 teaspoon peanut butter, 1 tablespoon raisins
- ■ 1 rib celery, 1 teaspoon peanut butter, 1 tablespoon raisins, 1 ounce turkey
- ● ½ to 1 rib celery, ½ to 1 teaspoon peanut butter, ½ to 1 tablespoon raisins

DINNER

Lean beef steak, succotash, side salad with olive oil vinaigrette

- ◆ 3 ounces steak, ½ cup succotash, 1 cup salad with 1 teaspoon olive oil and balsamic vinegar

- 4 ounces steak, 1 cup succotash, 1 cup salad with 1 teaspoon olive oil and balsamic vinegar

- 1 to 2 ounces steak, ¼ cup succotash, ¼ to ½ cup salad with ½ teaspoon olive oil and balsamic vinegar

Veggie burger, Baked French Fries made with sweet potatoes (page 255), steamed broccoli with low-fat Cheddar cheese

- 1 bun, 1 burger, 1 serving fries, broccoli with 1 ounce cheese

- 1 bun, 1 burger, 2 servings fries, broccoli with 1 ounce cheese

- ¼ to ½ bun, ¼ to ½ burger, ½ serving fries, broccoli with ½ to 1 ounce cheese

Soft tacos made with whole wheat tortillas, grilled steak or chicken, tomatoes, lettuce, grilled peppers, and low-fat cheese; milk

- 2 tortillas, 3 ounces meat, tomatoes, lettuce, and peppers, 1 ounce cheese, 1 cup fat-free milk

- 3 tortillas, 4 ounces meat, tomatoes, lettuce, and peppers, 1 ounce cheese, 1 cup fat-free milk

- 1 tortilla, 1 to 2 ounces meat, tomatoes, lettuce, and peppers, ½ to 1 ounce cheese, ½ to 1 cup low-fat milk

▼WEDNESDAY

Choose one option for each meal and snack.

BREAKFAST

Whole Wheat Pancakes (page 239), vegetarian or low-fat sausage

- 2 pancakes, 2 pieces sausage

- 3 pancakes, 3 pieces sausage

- 1 or 2 pancakes, 1 or 2 pieces sausage

Fruit Smoothie (page 263)

- ½ serving smoothie

- 1 serving smoothie, 2 tablespoons protein powder

- ¼ serving smoothie

Shrimp and Veggie Omelet (page 240) with whole grain toast

- 1 serving omelet, 1 slice toast

- 1 serving omelet, 1 slice toast

- ¼ to ½ serving omelet, ½ to 1 slice toast

SNACK

Low-fat cottage cheese with fresh cherries

- ¼ cup cottage cheese, ½ cup cherries

- ½ cup cottage cheese, ½ cup cherries

- 2 to 3 tablespoons cottage cheese, ¼ cup cherries

Crispbread dipped in cottage cheese mixed with cinnamon

- ◆ 3 crispbread, ¼ cup cottage cheese

- ■ 3 crispbread, ½ cup cottage cheese

- ● 1 to 2 crispbread, 2 to 3 tablespoons cottage cheese

Low-fat cheese and apple slices on whole grain crackers

- ◆ 1 ounce cheese, ½ apple, 3 crackers

- ■ 2 ounces cheese, ½ apple, 3 crackers

- ● ½ ounce cheese, ¼ apple, 2 to 3 crackers

LUNCH (EAT IN)

Small baked potato topped with chili, carrots

- ◆ 1 potato, ½ cup chili with 2 ounces lean meat, carrots

- ■ 1 potato, ½ cup chili with 3 ounces lean meat, carrots

- ● ½ potato, ¼ to ½ cup chili with 1 to 2 ounces lean meat, carrots

LUNCH (EAT OUT)

Wendy's Ultimate Chicken Grill sandwich, side salad with low-fat dressing

- ◆ ½ sandwich, salad with 1 tablespoon dressing

- ■ 1 sandwich, salad with 1 tablespoon dressing

- ● ¼ sandwich, ½ salad with ½ tablespoon dressing

LUNCH (AT SCHOOL)

Chicken Salad (page 244) on whole grain bread, cucumber slices, red grapes

- ◆ 1 slice bread, 1 serving chicken salad, cucumber slices, 15 grapes

- ■ 1 slice bread, 1 serving chicken salad, cucumber slices, 15 grapes

- ● ½ to 1 slice bread, ¼ to ½ serving chicken salad, cucumber slices, 6 to 10 grapes

SNACK

Protein bar (14+ grams protein, 25 grams carbohydrates, less than 3 grams fat)

- ◆ ½ energy bar

- ■ 1 energy bar

- ● ¼ to ½ energy bar

Reduced-fat mozzarella sticks with kiwifruit

- ◆ 1 cheese stick, ½ kiwifruit

- ■ 1 cheese stick, 1 kiwifruit

- ● ½ to 1 cheese stick, ¼ to ½ kiwifruit

White bean dip with small toasted whole wheat pita

- ◆ ¼ cup dip, 1 pita

- ■ ¼ cup dip, 1 pita

- ● 2 tablespoons dip, ½ pita

DINNER

Roasted chicken, steamed green beans, brown rice casserole with low-fat Cheddar cheese and steamed spinach, milk

- ◆ 3 ounces chicken, green beans, ⅓ cup rice with 1 ounce cheese, spinach, 1 cup fat-free milk

- ■ 4 ounces chicken, green beans, ⅓ cup rice with 1 ounce cheese, spinach, 1 cup fat-free milk

- ● 1 to 2 ounces chicken, green beans, ⅓ cup rice with 1 ounce cheese, spinach, ½ to 1 cup low-fat milk

Feta-Stuffed Chicken (page 247), side salad with olive oil vinaigrette

- ◆ ¾ serving chicken, 1 cup salad with 1 teaspoon olive oil and balsamic vinegar

- ■ 1 serving chicken, 1 cup salad with 1 teaspoon olive oil and balsamic vinegar

- ● ¼ to ½ serving chicken, ¼ to ½ cup salad with ½ to 1 teaspoon olive oil and balsamic vinegar

Grilled Beef Tenderloin (page 249), baked potato with sour cream, Roasted Asparagus (page 258), milk

- ◆ ½ serving beef, 1 small potato with 1 tablespoon sour cream, 1 serving asparagus, 1 cup fat-free milk

- ■ ½ serving beef, 1 large potato with 1 tablespoon sour cream, 1 serving asparagus, 1 cup fat-free milk

- ● ¾ serving beef, ½ small potato with ½ tablespoon sour cream, ½ serving asparagus, ½ to 1 cup low-fat milk

▼THURSDAY

Choose one option for each meal and snack.

BREAKFAST

High-fiber, high-protein cereal with milk

- ◆ ½ cup cereal, 3 tablespoons protein powder, 1 cup fat-free milk

- ■ 1 cup cereal, 3 tablespoons protein powder, 1 cup fat-free milk

- ● ½ to 1 cup cereal, ½ to 1 cup low-fat milk

Breakfast Sandwich (page 237)

- ◆ 1 sandwich

- ■ 1 sandwich, 1 piece fruit

- ● ½ sandwich

French toast made with whole grain bread, low-fat or vegetarian sausage

- ◆ 2 slices French toast, 1 piece sausage

- ■ 3 slices French toast, 2 pieces sausage

- ● ½ to 1 piece French toast, 1 piece sausage

SNACK

Low-fat Cheddar cheese on small whole wheat pita, apple

- ◆ 1 ounce cheese, ½ pita, ½ apple

- ■ 1 ounce cheese, ½ pita, ½ apple

- ● ½ ounce cheese, ½ pita, ¼ apple

One-half peanut butter and jelly sandwich with sliced strawberries (with natural peanut butter and all-fruit jam)

- ◆ ½ slice bread, ½ teaspoon peanut butter, ½ teaspoon jam, ¼ cup strawberries

- ■ 1 slice bread, 1 teaspoon peanut butter, 1 teaspoon jam, ¼ cup strawberries

- ● ½ slice bread, ½ teaspoon peanut butter, ½ teaspoon jam, 2 to 3 tablespoons strawberries

LUNCH (EAT IN)

Baked potato with steamed broccoli and low-fat Cheddar cheese, milk

- ◆ 1 small potato, broccoli, 1 ounce cheese, 1 cup fat-free milk

- ■ 1 medium potato, broccoli, 2 ounces cheese, 1 cup fat-free milk

- ● ½ small potato, broccoli, ½ to 1 ounce cheese, ½ to 1 cup low-fat milk

LUNCH (EAT OUT)

Boston Market rotisserie turkey, vegetable medley, sweet corn

- ◆ 2 ounces turkey, 1 cup vegetables, ½ cup corn

- ■ 3 ounces turkey, 1 cup vegetables, 1 cup corn

- ● 1 to 2 ounces turkey, ¼ to ½ cup vegetables, ¼ cup corn

LUNCH (AT SCHOOL)

Roast beef sandwich on whole grain bread, side salad with olive oil vinaigrette, cantaloupe cubes

- ◆ 1 slice bread, 2 ounces roast beef, 1 cup salad with 1 teaspoon olive oil and balsamic vinegar, 1 cup cantaloupe cubes

- ■ 2 slices bread, 3 ounces roast beef, 1 cup salad with 1 teaspoon olive oil and balsamic vinegar, 1 cup cantaloupe cubes

- ● 1 slice bread, 1 to 2 ounces roast beef, ½ cup salad with ½ teaspoon olive oil and balsamic vinegar, ¼ to ½ cup cantaloupe cubes

SNACK

Apple Ladybug Treats (page 260)

- ◆ 1 serving treats, 1 ounce ham

- ■ 1 serving treats, 2 ounces ham

- ● 1 serving treats

Turkey and tomato slices on small whole grain bagel with lemon pepper

- ◆ 1 ounce turkey, tomato, ½ bagel

- ■ 2 ounces turkey, tomato, 1 bagel

- ½ to 1 ounce turkey, tomato slices, ¼ to ½ bagel

Fruit Smoothie (page 263)

- ◆ ½ serving smoothie

- ■ 1 serving smoothie, 2 tablespoons protein powder

- ● ¼ serving smoothie

DINNER

Grilled lean steak, Roasted Vegetables (page 258), milk

- ◆ 3 ounces steak, 1 serving vegetables, 1 cup fat-free milk

- ■ 4 ounces steak, 1 serving vegetables, 1 cup fat-free milk

- ● 2 to 3 ounces steak, ½ to 1 serving vegetables, ½ to 1 cup low-fat milk

Grilled Salmon (page 245), Wild Rice Casserole (page 254), green beans

- ◆ 1 serving salmon, 1 serving casserole, green beans

- ■ 1 serving salmon, 1½ servings casserole, green beans

- ● ½ serving salmon, ¼ to ½ serving casserole, green beans

Baked chicken strips, Baked French Fries (page 255), steamed cauliflower sprinkled with low-fat cheese

- ◆ 3 ounces chicken, 1 serving fries, cauliflower with 1 ounce cheese

- ■ 4 ounces chicken, 2 servings fries, cauliflower with 1 ounce cheese

- ● 1 to 2 ounces chicken, ¼ to ½ serving fries, cauliflower with ½ ounce cheese

▼ FRIDAY

Choose one option for each meal and snack.

BREAKFAST

Low-fat cheese melted on whole grain toast

- ◆ 2 ounces cheese, 2 slices toast

- ■ 2 ounces cheese, 2 slices toast, 1 cup fat-free milk

- ● 1 ounce cheese, ½ to 1 slice toast

Scrambled egg with whole grain toast

- ◆ 1 egg and 1 egg white, 2 slices toast

- ■ 1 egg and 2 egg whites, 3 slices toast

- ● 1 egg, 1 slice toast

French toast made with whole grain bread, low-fat or vegetarian sausage

- ◆ 2 slices French toast, 1 piece sausage

- ■ 3 slices French toast, 2 pieces sausage

- ● ½ to 1 slice French toast, 1 piece sausage

SNACK

Fun Fruit Kebabs (page 263) dipped in low-fat vanilla yogurt

- ◆ 1 kebab, ½ cup yogurt

- ■ 1 kebab, ½ cup yogurt mixed with ¼ cup cottage cheese

- ● ½ to 1 kebab, ¼ to ½ cup yogurt

Turkey and low-fat cheese on whole grain crackers, dried apricots

- ◆ ½ ounce turkey, ½ ounce cheese, 3 crackers, 2 apricots

- ■ 1 ounce turkey, 1 ounce cheese, 3 crackers, 2 apricots

- ● ½ ounce turkey, ½ ounce cheese, 2 crackers, 1 apricot

Low-fat cottage cheese with fresh pineapple and almonds

- ◆ ¼ cup cottage cheese, ½ cup pineapple, 8 almonds

- ■ ½ cup cottage cheese, 1 cup pineapple, 8 almonds

- ● 2 to 3 tablespoons cottage cheese, ¼ cup pineapple, 3 or 4 almonds

LUNCH (EAT IN)

Tuna casserole with whole wheat angel hair pasta, shredded low-fat Cheddar cheese, steamed broccoli, milk

- ◆ 2 ounces tuna, ½ cup pasta, 1 ounce cheese, broccoli, 1 cup fat-free milk

- ■ 3 ounces tuna, 1 cup pasta, 1 ounce cheese, broccoli, 1 cup fat-free milk

- ● 1 to 2 ounces tuna, ¼ cup pasta, ½ ounce cheese, broccoli, ½ to 1 cup low-fat milk

LUNCH (EAT OUT)

Thin-crust pizza with vegetables, chicken, and reduced-fat mozzarella cheese; side salad with olive oil vinaigrette

- ◆ 1 slice pizza with vegetables, 1 ounce chicken, 1 ounce cheese, 1 cup salad with 1 teaspoon olive oil and balsamic vinegar

- ■ 1 slice pizza with vegetables, 2 ounces chicken, 1 ounce cheese, 1 cup salad with 1 teaspoon olive oil and balsamic vinegar

- ● ¼ to ½ slice pizza with vegetables, 1 ounce chicken, 1 ounce cheese, ¼ to ½ cup salad with ½ to 1 teaspoon olive oil and balsamic vinegar

LUNCH (AT SCHOOL)

Peanut butter and banana sandwich on whole grain bread (with natural peanut butter), milk

- ◆ 1 slice bread, 1 teaspoon peanut butter, ½ banana, 1 cup fat-free milk

- ■ 1 slice bread, 1 teaspoon peanut butter, ½ banana, 1 cup fat-free milk

- ● ½ slice bread, ½ teaspoon peanut butter, ¼ banana, ½ to 1 cup low-fat milk

SNACK

Ham sandwich with fresh tomato on whole grain bread

- ◆ 1 slice bread, 1 ounce ham, tomato slices

- ■ 1 slice bread, 2 ounces ham, tomato slices

- ● ½ to 1 slice bread, 1 ounce ham, tomato slices

Veggie Dip (page 262) with fresh-cut vegetables

- ◆ 1 serving dip, vegetables

- ■ 2 servings dip, vegetables

- ● ½ serving dip, vegetables

Zesty Tuna Salad (page 242) on whole grain crackers, apple

- ◆ ¼ serving tuna, 3 crackers, ½ apple

- ■ ½ serving tuna, 6 crackers, ½ apple

- ● ¼ serving tuna, 2 or 3 crackers, ¼ apple

DINNER

Chicken or tofu stir-fry with broccoli, water chestnuts, and carrots; brown rice; milk

- ◆ 3 ounces chicken or tofu with vegetables, ⅓ cup rice, 1 cup fat-free milk

- ■ 4 ounces chicken or tofu with vegetables, ⅔ cup rice, 1 cup fat-free milk

- ● 2 to 3 ounces chicken or tofu with vegetables, 2 to 4 tablespoons rice, ½ to 1 cup low-fat milk

Roast chicken, Wild Rice Casserole (page 254), Broccoli, Orange, and Watercress Salad (page 257)

- ◆ 3 ounces chicken, ½ serving casserole, 1 serving salad

- ■ 4 ounces chicken, 1 serving casserole, 1 serving salad

- ● 1 to 2 ounces chicken, ¼ to ½ serving casserole, ¼ to ½ serving salad

Stuffed Peppers (page 251), small whole grain roll, side salad with chicken and olive oil vinaigrette

- ◆ 1 serving peppers, 1 roll, 1 cup salad with 3 ounces chicken and 1 teaspoon olive oil and balsamic vinegar

- ■ 1 serving peppers, 1 roll, 1 cup salad with 4 ounces chicken and 1 teaspoon olive oil and balsamic vinegar

- ● ¼ to ½ serving peppers, 1 roll, ¼ cup salad with 1 to 2 ounces chicken and 1 teaspoon olive oil and balsamic vinegar

Choose one option for each meal and snack.

BREAKFAST

Ham and Vegetable Frittata (page 238) with whole grain toast

◆ 1 serving frittata, 1 slice toast

■ 1½ servings frittata, 1 slice toast

● ½ serving frittata, ½ slice toast

Whole Wheat Pancakes (page 239), low-fat or vegetarian sausage

◆ 2 pancakes, 2 pieces sausage

■ 3 pancakes, 3 pieces sausage

● 1 or 2 pancakes, 1 or 2 pieces sausage

High-fiber, high-protein cereal with milk

◆ ½ cup cereal, 3 tablespoons protein powder, 1 cup fat-free milk

■ 1 cup cereal, 3 tablespoons protein powder, 1 cup fat-free milk

● ½ to 1 cup cereal, ½ to 1 cup low-fat milk

SNACK

Hummus and fresh vegetables

◆ 4 tablespoons hummus, vegetables

■ 6 tablespoons hummus, vegetables

● 2 tablespoons hummus, vegetables

Low-fat cheese on whole grain crackers, apple slices

◆ 1 ounce cheese, 3 crackers, ½ apple

■ 1 ounce cheese, 6 crackers, ½ apple

● ½ ounce cheese, 2 or 3 crackers, ¼ apple

Low-fat yogurt with orange slices

◆ 1 cup yogurt, ½ orange

■ 1½ cups yogurt, 1 orange

● ½ to 1 cup yogurt, ¼ to ½ orange

LUNCH (EAT IN)

Wild Rice Apple Salad (page 255), grilled chicken

◆ ½ serving salad, 2 ounces chicken

■ 1 serving salad, 3 ounces chicken

● ¼ serving salad, 1 ounce chicken

Creamy Cauliflower Soup (page 244), small whole grain roll, salad with olive oil vinaigrette

◆ ¾ serving soup, 1 roll, 1 cup salad with 1 teaspoon olive oil and balsamic vinegar

■ 1 serving soup, 1 roll, 1 cup salad with 1 teaspoon olive oil and balsamic vinegar

● ¼ to ½ serving soup, 1 roll, ¼ to ½ cup salad with ½ teaspoon olive oil and balsamic vinegar

LUNCH (EAT OUT)

Spring roll, chicken vegetable soup

- ◆ 1 spring roll, 1 cup soup (with 2 ounces chicken), vegetables

- ◼ 1 spring roll, 1 cup soup (with 3 ounces chicken), vegetables

- ● ½ spring roll, ½ cup soup (with 1 to 2 ounces chicken), vegetables

SNACK

Apple slices with thinly spread peanut butter

- ◆ 1 apple, 1 teaspoon peanut butter

- ◼ 1 apple, 1 teaspoon peanut butter, 1 ounce turkey

- ● ¼ to ½ apple, ½ to 1 teaspoon peanut butter

Low-fat cottage cheese mixed with low-fat sour cream and sprinkled with cinnamon and brown sugar, with fresh fruit for dipping

- ◆ ¼ cup cottage cheese, 1 tablespoon sour cream, ½ cup fruit

- ◼ ½ cup cottage cheese, 1 tablespoon sour cream, ½ cup fruit

- ● 2 to 3 tablespoons cottage cheese, ½ tablespoon sour cream, ¼ cup fruit

Fresh Homemade Salsa (page 260) with baked chips

- ◆ Salsa, 6 chips

- ◼ Salsa, 12 chips

- ● Salsa, 4 to 6 chips

DINNER

Lean beef steak, corn, wild rice, steamed broccoli

- ◆ 3 ounces beef, ½ cup corn, ⅓ cup rice, broccoli

- ◼ 4 ounces beef, ½ cup corn, ⅓ cup rice, broccoli

- ● 1 to 2 ounces beef, 2 to 3 tablespoons corn, 2 to 3 tablespoons rice, broccoli

Quick and Spicy Fish Fillets (page 246), brown rice pilaf, Green Beans with Toasted Almonds (page 259), milk

- ◆ 1 serving fish, ⅓ cup pilaf, 1 serving green beans, 1 cup fat-free milk

- ◼ 1 serving fish, ⅔ cup pilaf, 1 serving green beans, 1 cup fat-free milk

- ● ½ serving fish, 3 to 4 tablespoons pilaf, ½ serving green beans, ½ to 1 cup low-fat milk

Chicken Vegetable Stew (page 248), small whole grain roll, side salad with olive oil vinaigrette

- ◆ 1 serving stew, 1 roll, 1 cup side salad with 1 teaspoon olive oil and balsamic vinegar

- ◼ 1 serving stew, 1 roll, 1 cup side salad with 1 teaspoon olive oil and balsamic vinegar

- ● ¼ to ½ serving stew, 1 roll, ¼ to ½ cup side salad with ½ teaspoon olive oil and balsamic vinegar

Choose one option for each meal and snack.

BREAKFAST

Whole Wheat Pancakes (page 239), low-fat or vegetarian sausage

♦ 2 pancakes, 2 pieces sausage

■ 3 pancakes, 3 pieces sausage

● 1 or 2 pancakes, 1 or 2 pieces sausage

Spinach and Feta Omelet (page 238)

♦ 1 serving omelet

■ 1 serving omelet

● ¼ to ½ serving omelet

Oatmeal with milk

♦ ½ cup oatmeal, 1 tablespoon protein powder, 1 cup fat-free milk

■ 1 cup oatmeal, 2 tablespoons protein powder, 1 cup fat-free milk

● ½ to 1 cup oatmeal, ½ to 1 cup low-fat milk

SNACK

Low-fat Jarlsberg cheese on whole grain toast, grapes

♦ 1 ounce cheese, ½ slice toast, 15 grapes

■ 2 ounces cheese, 1 slice toast, 15 grapes

● ½ to 1 ounce cheese, ½ slice toast, 6 to 10 grapes

Fun Fruit Kebabs (page 263) dipped in low-fat yogurt

♦ 1 kebab, ½ cup yogurt

■ 1 kebab, ½ cup yogurt mixed with ¼ cup cottage cheese

● ½ to 1 kebab, ¼ to ½ cup yogurt

Hard-cooked egg on whole grain toast

♦ 1 egg, 1 slice toast

■ 1 egg and 1 egg white, 1 slice toast

● ½ egg, ½ slice toast

LUNCH (EAT IN)

Veggie burger on whole wheat bun with lettuce and tomato, baby carrots, grapes

♦ 1 bun, 1 burger, lettuce and tomato, carrots, 15 grapes

■ 1 bun, 1 burger, lettuce and tomato, carrots, 15 grapes, 1 cup fat-free milk

● ½ bun, ¼ to ½ burger, lettuce and tomato, carrots, 6 to 10 grapes

Tomato soup, whole grain crackers, baby carrots

♦ 1 cup soup (made with fat-free milk), 6 crackers, carrots

■ 1½ cups soup (made with fat-free milk), 8 crackers, carrots

● ½ cup soup (made with low-fat milk), 3 to 6 crackers, carrots

LUNCH (EAT OUT)

Grilled chicken sandwich on whole grain bun, steamed vegetables

- ◆ 1 bun, 2 ounces chicken, vegetables

- ■ 1 bun, 3 ounces chicken, vegetables, 1 apple

- ● ½ bun, 1 to 2 ounces chicken, vegetables

SNACK

Veggie Dip (page 262) with fresh-cut vegetables

- ◆ 1 serving dip, vegetables

- ■ 2 servings dip, vegetables

- ● ½ serving dip, vegetables

Celery with thinly spread peanut butter topped with raisins

- ◆ 1 rib celery, 1 teaspoon peanut butter, 1 tablespoon raisins

- ■ 1 rib celery, 1 teaspoon peanut butter, 1 tablespoon raisins, 1 ounce turkey

- ● ½ to 1 rib celery, ½ to 1 teaspoon peanut butter, ½ to 1 tablespoon raisins

Low-fat cottage cheese with fresh cherries

- ◆ ¼ cup cottage cheese, ½ cup cherries

- ■ ½ cup cottage cheese, ½ cup cherries

- ● 2 to 3 tablespoons cottage cheese, ¼ cup cherries

DINNER

Feta-Stuffed Chicken (page 247), side salad with olive oil vinaigrette

- ◆ 1 serving chicken, 1 cup salad with 1 teaspoon olive oil and balsamic vinegar

- ■ 1 serving chicken, 1 cup salad with 1 teaspoon olive oil and balsamic vinegar

- ● ¼ to ½ serving chicken, ¼ to ½ cup salad with ½ teaspoon olive oil and balsamic vinegar

Roasted skinless chicken breast, red potatoes, steamed cabbage, milk

- ◆ 3 ounces chicken, ½ cup potatoes, ½ cup cabbage, 1 cup fat-free milk

- ■ 4 ounces chicken, 1 cup potatoes, ½ cup cabbage, 1 cup fat-free milk

- ● 1 to 2 ounces chicken, ¼ cup potatoes, ¼ cup cabbage, ½ to 1 cup low-fat milk

Grilled Beef Tenderloin (page 249), baked potato with low-fat sour cream, Roasted Asparagus (page 258), milk

- ◆ ½ serving beef, 1 small potato with 1 tablespoon sour cream, 1 serving asparagus, 1 cup fat-free milk

- ■ ½ serving beef, 1 large potato with 1 tablespoon sour cream, 1 serving asparagus, 1 cup fat-free milk

- ● ¼ serving beef, ½ small potato with ½ tablespoon sour cream, ½ serving asparagus, ½ to 1 cup low-fat milk

FITNESS FOCUS

Can you believe it? We are already at Week 6. You and your family members are 6 for 6! Just think about all that you have done to manage your fitness levels and body weight, without it taking over your daily schedules or depriving you of delicious food. Now you can take some of that fitness knowledge and help yourself and your family have a little fun by designing a weekly activity and circuit routine that each of you finds enjoyable, effective, and exactly what you want to do. First, a quick review.

WEEK	FITNESS FOCUS
1	Cardiovascular activities
2	Strength training
3	Core movements
4	Flexibility through stretching
5	Interval training

Week 6: Create Your Own Circuit Routines

Okay, your turn. Using the "buffet" of exercise from the first 5 weeks, it's time to be creative! Take a blank exercise/activity journal page and begin to build your own personal fitness routine!

Remember to use only my recommended exercises and activities for each age group. Make changes only with both your doctor's approval and that of a reputable health professional.

Step 1: Start with the cardiovascular activity of your choice for the recommended amount of time. Jot it down. (Do more time if you feel comfortable.)

Step 2: Add your strength-training activities. You can start from low-numbered exercises and progress to high numbers, or go from high to low. It's your choice—either way, the routine is still healthy, safe, and balanced.

Step 3: Add core movements from Week 3 and change as often as you like.

Step 4: Add just a few minutes of stretching—always.

Step 5: Challenge yourself and have fun as you add intervals of cardiovascular activity and sports-specific movements. (Always start with shorter time intervals and add more when you feel comfortable.)

Make sure you write it down so you can keep track of what you actually do in Week 6 just as you've done in previous weeks.

FIT FAMILY ACTIVITY

In the last of our 6 weeks of family activities, I want to offer you and your family an idea that combines activity with celebration. Why not? You all deserve it. You have worked hard as you have adopted a new lifestyle that will afford you good health for many years to come.

My Week 6 Fit Family Activity suggestion is an active weekend getaway for everyone at a special place. Now, this in itself could be challenging, since we all have different ideas of what and where a special place can be. But let's home in on this idea. Depending on your budget, you can either travel out of state or stay close to home. I'm thinking about a hotel destination where there will be lots of active choices that will satisfy everyone. It could be a big theme park or a hotel around the corner with an outdoor or indoor pool. Regardless of where it is and whether you take a plane, train, car, or bus to get there, try to schedule a weekend away from home at a destination that has lots of opportunities for activity.

Do a little research and call around to find out what accommodations, services, amenities, and activities are offered. In this day and age, the hotel and resort industry has become very family friendly. Many have "kids' fun weekends," with all kinds of great sports and activities.

Ask about hiking trails where you and your family can have a healthy picnic, climb a mountainside, or trek to a waterfall. Ask about horseback or pony riding lessons and trails. Many resorts have pools, basketball and tennis courts, batting cages, driving ranges, and golf courses.

Perhaps you can go on an afternoon bike ride, canoe trip, or other activity—it doesn't matter what. Just do it together, make it healthy, and have fun.

There's just one catch: You'll have to take me along to make sure everything is going smoothly. I can go, can't I? No? Well, at least send me a postcard!

You could have all this fun together halfway across the country or close to home. It doesn't matter, as long as you make it clear that rewards can be earned in a healthy home.

WEEK 6 FINAL THOUGHTS

Hey, Mom, I am really very proud of you and excited that you are reading these words 6 weeks after we started this journey together. You and your family have worked through a lot together and hopefully have had fun. This is a big week for you, and I want everyone to remain focused. Go celebrate a little, but remember, you are still working together and striving to hit some important goals. Nothing will stop you from reaching them!

WEEK 6 ACTION STEP SUMMARY

❑ Review goals—recommit if needed and make adjustments.
❑ Review food diaries and exercise/activity journals—take a look at how your eating habits have improved over the past 6 weeks.
❑ Prepare weekly meal plans—Food Focus: dining out.
❑ Fitness Focus: Design your own routine.
❑ Fit Family Activity: Congratulate yourselves with an active family weekend!

GREAT JOB!

As you are now reading my final words, keep this in mind: This book should not be put away on an unreachable bookshelf. Keep it somewhere accessible. You are now the coach; you are now in full control, armed with all the knowledge and experience that you need to know regarding health and fitness well-being. You have taken this project from the very beginning, embraced it, and worked it into the lives of your loved ones. It hasn't been easy—it never is—but you did it! I have worked with many families and have seen the struggles and challenges along the way, and I've fine-tuned their feedback and experiences in order to present it to you within this book. You and your family can now live the rest of your lives with good health. More important, you now have the know-how to maintain that good health at any time, any age, and anywhere you may live on this earth.

APPENDIX A

Our Fabulous Family Recipes

▼ BREAKFAST

BREAKFAST SANDWICH

4 servings

- 4   egg whites
- 4   vegetarian sausage patties or lean turkey sausage patties
- 4   whole wheat English muffins
- 4   ounces low-fat Cheddar cheese

1. Heat a medium skillet over medium heat. Coat with cooking spray and fry the egg whites and sausage.

2. Toast the English muffins and assemble the egg whites, sausage, and cheese on half of the muffin. Add the top and enjoy.

Per serving: 290 calories, 22 g protein, 30 g carbohydrates, 10 g fat, 4 g fiber

HAM AND VEGETABLE FRITTATA

4 servings

1	teaspoon olive oil	4	ounces ham, chopped
4	egg whites	½	tomato, chopped
2	eggs		Salt and ground black pepper to taste
4	cups mixed vegetables (such as broccoli, ¼ cup onions, green or red bell peppers), lightly steamed		

1. Preheat the oven to 350°F. Lightly coat a 9" glass pie pan with olive oil.

2. In a large bowl, whisk the egg whites and eggs until foamy. Add the vegetables, ham, and tomato.

3. Pour the mixture into the pie pan and bake for about 15 minutes, or until set. Loosen the edges with a spatula, slice, and season with the salt and pepper.

Per serving: 150 calories, 13 g protein, 6 g carbohydrates, 9 g fat, 3 g fiber

SPINACH AND FETA OMELET

2 servings

4	egg whites	2	ounces feta cheese
2	eggs	1	cup fresh spinach, chopped

1. Heat a medium skillet over medium heat and coat with cooking spray.

2. In a medium bowl, whisk the egg whites and eggs together, then pour into the skillet. With a rubber spatula, loosen the edges and allow the eggs to flow under as they cook.

3. When the eggs are mostly cooked but still slightly liquid on top, place the cheese and spinach on top.

4. Using a rubber spatula, fold the omelet in half. Allow the feta time to melt (approximately 1 minute) and serve.

Per serving: 210 calories, 16 g protein, 3 g carbohydrates, 14 g fat, 1 g fiber

WHOLE WHEAT PANCAKES

Makes about 12 pancakes

1½	cups whole wheat pastry flour		1⅓	cups low-fat milk
1	tablespoon granulated sugar		2	tablespoons vegetable oil
1½	teaspoons baking powder			Fresh berries (such as strawberries, blueberries, raspberries)
	Dash of salt			
2	eggs			Maple syrup or confectioners' sugar

1. In a large bowl, stir together the flour, granulated sugar, baking powder, salt, eggs, milk, and vegetable oil.

2. Coat a hot griddle with cooking spray. Pour on approximately ¼ cup batter per pancake. When bubbles begin to form, flip the pancakes. Remove from the griddle when cooked through.

3. Serve hot with the berries and top with the maple syrup or confectioners' sugar.

Per pancake: 125 calories, 4 g protein, 15 g carbohydrates, 3 g fat, 3 g fiber

Variations: To make Buttermilk Pancakes, substitute ½ teaspoon baking soda for the baking powder and buttermilk for the milk.

For Cornmeal Pancakes, decrease the flour to ¾ cup and add ¾ cup yellow cornmeal.

To make Blueberry Pancakes, gently fold 2 cups rinsed and drained fresh blueberries into the batter.

SHRIMP AND VEGGIE OMELET

4 servings

1	onion, chopped	½	cup 1% milk
1	clove garlic, crushed	1	teaspoon curry powder
½	cup sliced fresh mushrooms	1	tablespoon olive oil
¼	cup chopped green bell pepper	4	ounces shredded low-fat Cheddar cheese
12	medium shrimp, peeled and deveined	1	tomato, sliced
4	egg whites		Salt and ground black pepper to taste
2	eggs		

1. In a medium nonstick saucepan over medium heat, cook and stir the onion, garlic, mushrooms, and bell pepper until tender, about 5 minutes. Stir in the shrimp and cook until opaque. Remove from the heat and set aside.

2. In a medium bowl, beat together the egg whites, eggs, and milk. Stir in the curry powder.

3. Heat the oil in a medium saucepan over medium heat. Pour in the egg mixture and cook for 5 minutes, or until firm.

4. Top with the cheese, tomato, and the onion and shrimp mixture. Fold the eggs over the filling and serve warm. Season with the salt and pepper.

Per serving: 220 calories, 21 g protein, 8 g carbohydrates, 11 g fat, 1 g fiber

COUSCOUS WITH PORTOBELLO MUSHROOMS AND SUN-DRIED TOMATOES

4 servings

1	cup dehydrated sun-dried tomatoes	⅓	cup fresh basil or ¼ teaspoon dried
½	package (10 ounces) couscous	¼	cup fresh cilantro, chopped
1	teaspoon olive oil		Juice of ½ lemon (about 2 tablespoons)
3	cloves garlic, pressed		Salt and ground black pepper to taste
1	bunch green onions, chopped (about 1 cup)	4	ounces portobello mushroom caps, sliced

1. Place the tomatoes in a bowl with 1 cup water. Soak for 30 minutes, or until rehydrated. Drain, reserving the water, and chop.

2. In a medium saucepan, combine the reserved tomato water with enough water to yield 1½ cups. Bring to a boil and stir in the couscous. Cover, remove from the heat, and let stand for 5 minutes, or until the liquid has been absorbed. Gently fluff with a fork.

3. Heat the oil in a large skillet. Stir in the tomatoes, garlic, and onions. Cook and stir for about 5 minutes, or until the onions are tender. Add the basil, cilantro, and lemon juice. Season with the salt and pepper. Add the mushrooms and continue cooking for 3 to 5 minutes. Toss with the cooked couscous and serve.

Per serving: 120 calories, 5 g protein, 24 g carbohydrates, 1 g fat, 4 g fiber

EGG SALAD

4 servings

8	eggs	1	teaspoon ground paprika
1	tablespoon low-fat mayonnaise	½	red onion, minced
2	tablespoons Dijon mustard		Salt and ground black pepper to taste
1	teaspoon dried dillweed		

1. Place the eggs in a medium saucepan and cover with cold water. Bring to a boil, then cover, remove from the heat, and let stand for 10 to 12 minutes. Remove the eggs, cool, peel, and chop.

2. In a large bowl, combine the eggs, mayonnaise, mustard, dillweed, paprika, and onion. Mash well with a fork or wooden spoon. Season with the salt and pepper. Serve on bread as a sandwich or over crisp lettuce as a salad.

Per serving: 191 calories, 13 g protein, 4 g carbohydrates, 13 g fat, 1 g fiber

ZESTY TUNA SALAD

2 servings

1	can (6 ounces) tuna, drained	1	rib celery, chopped
1	teaspoon low-fat mayonnaise	¼	cup chopped onion
1	teaspoon sweet pickle relish	¼	teaspoon ground black pepper
1	teaspoon Dijon mustard		

1. Mash the tuna in a small bowl with a fork. Add the mayonnaise, relish, mustard, celery, onion, and pepper and stir to combine. Chill and serve.

Per serving: 132 calories, 22 g protein, 4 g carbohydrates, 3 g fat, 1 g fiber

VEGETABLE SANDWICH

1 serving

2	slices whole grain bread	1	ounce provolone cheese
1	tablespoon Dijon mustard	2	tablespoons fresh basil
2	slices tomato	3	slices red onion
2	tablespoons alfalfa sprouts	½	red bell pepper, roasted

1. Toast the bread, if desired, and spread with the mustard. Layer the tomato, sprouts, cheese, basil, onion, and pepper on one slice of the bread and top with the second slice.

Per serving: 200 calories, 8 g protein, 38 g carbohydrates, 3 g fat, 7 g fiber

TURKEY APPLE SANDWICH

1 serving

2	slices whole grain bread	3	ounces smoked turkey breast
1	tablespoon low-fat mayonnaise	2	leaves Romaine lettuce
2	slices Granny Smith apple		

1. Toast the bread, if desired, and spread with the mayonnaise. Assemble the apple, turkey, and lettuce on one slice of the bread and top with the second slice.

Per serving: 300 calories, 22 g protein, 35 g carbohydrates, 8 g fat, 5 g fiber

CHICKEN SALAD

4 servings

1½ cups chopped, cooked skinless chicken breast	⅓ cup low-fat mayonnaise
½ cup chopped celery	2 teaspoons Dijon mustard
¼ cup thinly sliced green or yellow onion	

1. In a large bowl, stir together the chicken, celery, onion, mayonnaise, and mustard. Chill and serve on whole grain bread or Romaine lettuce with sliced tomatoes and cucumbers.

Per serving: 160 calories, 16 g protein, 3 g carbohydrates, 9 g fat, 1 g fiber

Note: One leaf of lettuce, 2 slices of tomato, and a 1" slice of cucumber will add 25 calories and 0.5 gram of fiber to the recipe.

CREAMY CAULIFLOWER SOUP

4 servings

1 pound fresh cauliflower florets	½ teaspoon ground black pepper
4 medium potatoes, peeled and cubed	½ teaspoon salt
1 large onion, chopped	½ teaspoon hot sauce
3 cups chicken broth	2 teaspoons dried thyme leaves
2 cups 1% milk	

1. Place the cauliflower in a large saucepan, cover with water, and bring to a boil. Reduce the heat and simmer until barely tender. Drain.

2. Add the potatoes, onion, broth, milk, pepper, salt, and hot sauce and return to a simmer. Cook for about 20 minutes, or until the vegetables are fully cooked. Remove from the heat.

3. Place 1 to 2 cups of hot soup in a blender and puree at low speed until smooth. Pour into a separate container. Repeat with the remaining soup.

Per serving: 250 calories, 11 g protein, 49 g carbohydrates, 2 g fat, 9 g fiber

HOMEMADE PITA PIZZAS

4 servings

1	cup pizza sauce	8	large mushrooms, sliced
4	large whole wheat pitas	1	large tomato, sliced
6	ounces reduced-fat mozzarella, shredded	6	ounces cooked boneless, skinless chicken breast, cut into bite-size pieces
½	cup chopped broccoli		

1. Preheat the oven to 350°F.

2. Spread the pizza sauce on the pitas. Top with the cheese, broccoli, mushrooms, tomato, and chicken, divided evenly among the pitas.

3. Place on a baking sheet and bake for 15 minutes.

Per serving: 300 calories, 19 g protein, 40 g carbohydrates, 8 g fat, 6 g fiber

GRILLED SALMON

6 servings

1½	pounds salmon fillets	⅓	cup soy sauce
½	teaspoon lemon pepper	⅓	cup brown sugar
½	teaspoon garlic powder	⅓	cup water
¼	teaspoon salt		

1. Season the salmon with the lemon pepper, garlic powder, and salt.

2. In a small bowl, stir together the soy sauce, brown sugar, and water until the sugar is dissolved. Place the fish in a large resealable plastic bag with the soy sauce mixture. Seal and turn to coat. Refrigerate for at least 2 hours.

3. Lightly oil the grill rack. Preheat the grill to medium.

4. Place the salmon on the grill and discard the marinade. Cook for 6 to 8 minutes per side, or until the fish flakes easily with a fork.

Per serving: 214 calories, 23 g protein, 13 g carbohydrates, 7 g fat, 0 g fiber

QUICK AND SPICY FISH FILLETS

6 servings

6	fine-textured fish fillets (such as flounder, sole, or cod), 4 ounces each	½	cup cornflake crumbs
½	cup grated Parmesan cheese	¼	teaspoon ground red pepper
		1	egg, beaten

1. Preheat the oven to 450°F. Oil or grease a shallow baking dish.

2. In a shallow bowl, combine the cheese, crumbs, and red pepper. Dip the fish in the egg, then into the cheese mixture, coating evenly.

3. Place the fish in the baking dish. Bake for 5 to 10 minutes, or until the fish flakes easily with a fork.

Per serving: 200 calories, 23 g protein, 3 g carbohydrates, 7 g fat, 0 g fiber

Variation: Substitute boneless, skinless chicken breast halves for the fish. Decrease the oven temperature to 400°F. Bake for 15 to 20 minutes, or until the chicken is cooked through.

SWEET POTATO MINESTRONE

10 servings

1	tablespoon vegetable oil	1	large sweet potato, peeled and chopped
1	large onion, chopped	2	large carrots, thinly sliced
2	large ribs celery, chopped	1	cup green beans, cut into 1" pieces
2½	teaspoons Italian seasoning	5	cloves garlic, minced
1	can (28 ounces) Italian-style diced tomatoes		Salt and ground black pepper to taste
2½	cups vegetable broth		

1. Heat the oil in a soup pot over medium-high heat. Sauté the onion, celery, and seasoning until tender, about 5 minutes. Stir in the tomatoes (with juice), broth, sweet potatoes, carrots, green beans, and garlic. Bring to a boil, then reduce the heat to low and simmer, stirring occasionally, for about 30 minutes, or until the vegetables are tender. Season with the salt and pepper.

Per serving: 147 calories, 5 g protein, 26 g carbohydrates, 3 g fat, 5 g fiber

FETA-STUFFED CHICKEN

4 servings

4	boneless, skinless chicken breast halves, 4 ounces each	3	cups fresh spinach
¼	cup dried bread crumbs	½	cup chopped fresh basil
¼	cup crumbled feta cheese with basil and tomato	1	tablespoon balsamic vinegar
2	teaspoons olive oil	1	teaspoon olive oil
			Ground black pepper to taste

1. Preheat the oven to 400°F. Coat an 8" square baking dish with cooking spray.

2. Place each chicken breast half between 2 sheets of heavy-duty plastic wrap and flatten to ¼" thickness with a meat mallet or rolling pin. Dredge the chicken in the bread crumbs, then spoon 1 tablespoon of the cheese onto each piece and fold in half.

3. Place the chicken in the baking dish and drizzle with the olive oil. Bake, uncovered, for 25 minutes, or until no longer pink.

4. In a medium bowl, combine the spinach and basil. Drizzle with the vinegar and oil and toss well. Serve the chicken over the salad, seasoned with the pepper.

Per serving: 207 calories, 30 g protein, 7 g carbohydrate, 6 g fat, 2 g fiber

CAJUN-SPICED CHICKEN

4 servings

½	cup all-purpose flour	4	boneless, skinless chicken breast halves, cut into strips
1	teaspoon Cajun seasoning	4	teaspoons olive oil
1	cup fat-free milk		

1. In a shallow plate or bowl, mix together the flour and seasoning. Pour the milk into a bowl and dip the chicken into it. Dredge the chicken in the flour mixture, coating evenly.

2. Heat the oil in a large skillet. Add the chicken and sauté until browned and crisp.

Per serving: 311 calories, 31 g protein, 16 g carbohydrates, 10 g fat, 1 g fiber

CHICKEN VEGETABLE STEW

4 servings

4	boneless, skinless chicken breast halves, cut into bite-size pieces	¼	teaspoon ground turmeric
1	onion, chopped	3	tablespoons tomato paste
½	pound baby carrots	½	cup water
4	potatoes, peeled and chopped	¼	teaspoon garlic powder (optional)
½	teaspoon salt	½	teaspoon ground black pepper (optional)

1. Place the chicken, onion, carrots, and potatoes in a large pot. Add the salt and turmeric. Dissolve the tomato paste in the water and stir into the stew. Add the garlic powder and pepper, if using. Cook for 1 to 1½ hours on medium-low heat.

Per serving: 270 calories, 31 g protein, 32 g carbohydrates, 2 g fat, 5 g fiber

BLACK BEAN SOUP

4 servings

10	sun-dried tomatoes	2	cans (16 ounces each) black beans, undrained
1	cup boiling water	1	tablespoon orange juice
2	tablespoons olive oil	1	tablespoon lemon juice
1	medium onion, minced	¼	teaspoon cumin
2	medium green or red bell peppers, chopped	1	jalapeno, minced and seeds removed, or
2	cloves garlic, minced		¼ teaspoon cayenne pepper
⅓	cup water		

1. In small bowl, cover the tomatoes with boiling water and soften for about 15 minutes.

2. Heat the oil in a medium saucepan. Add the onion, peppers, and garlic and sauté until soft.

3. Chop the softened, sun-dried tomatoes and add, along with water, to the vegetable mixture.

4. Add the remaining ingredients and heat through. Mash about ½ of the soup in the saucepan or remove ½, puree it in blender, and return it to the pan.

Per serving: 300 calories, 13 g protein, 43 g carbohydrates, 8 g fat, 13 g fiber

GRILLED BEEF TENDERLOIN

4 servings

1½ pounds beef tenderloin	2 tablespoons fresh tarragon, minced
1 tablespoon black peppercorns, crushed	

1. Preheat the grill or broiler.

2. Roll the beef in the pepper and tarragon.

3. Place the beef about 4" from the broiler or on foil on the grill rack. Cook for about 25 minutes, turning frequently with tongs. Let stand for 5 minutes before slicing.

Per serving: 220 calories, 27 g protein, 0 g carbohydrates, 11 g fat, 0 g fiber

CABBAGE ROLL-UPS

6 servings

12 cabbage leaves	½ teaspoon thyme
1½ pounds 95% lean ground turkey	1 can (28 ounces) tomato sauce or diced tomatoes
1 small onion, chopped	
1 cup brown rice, cooked	Salt and ground black pepper to taste

1. Steam the cabbage leaves until tender, about 10 minutes. Remove the hard inner core.

2. In a large skillet, brown the turkey and onion. Add the rice, thyme, salt, and pepper.

3. Pour a small amount of the tomato sauce in the bottom of a 13" × 9" baking dish.

4. Place equal portions of the meat mixture on each cabbage leaf. Fold in the sides of each leaf and roll up. Place the rolls, seam side down, on top of the tomato sauce in the baking dish.

5. Pour the remaining tomato sauce over the cabbage rolls, cover, and bake at 350°F for 30 minutes, or until bubbly. Season with the salt and pepper.

Per serving: 240 calories, 27 g protein, 18 g carbohydrates, 7 g fat, 3 g fiber

CHICKEN CREOLE

6 servings

2	pounds boneless, skinless chicken breasts, cut into strips
2	teaspoons olive oil
2	medium onions, chopped
1	green bell pepper, chopped
2	ribs celery, chopped
2	cloves garlic, minced
1	cup tomato juice or tomato juice cocktail
2	tomatoes, chopped
½	teaspoon cayenne pepper
2	cups brown rice, cooked

1. In a large skillet, brown the chicken in the oil.

2. Add the onions, green pepper, celery, and garlic and sauté until crisp-tender.

3. Add the tomato juice, tomatoes, and cayenne pepper. Cover and simmer for about 20 minutes. Serve over the rice.

Per serving: 280 calories, 32 g protein, 30 g carbohydrates, 5 g fat, 5 g fiber

BAKED FISH WITH VEGETABLES

4 servings

1	cup tomato sauce
1	cup chopped celery
½	cup chopped green bell pepper
½	cup chopped onion
⅓	cup chopped carrots
2	tablespoons lemon juice
½	tablespoon salt
1	pound halibut fillets

1. In a small saucepan, combine the tomato sauce, celery, pepper, onion, carrots, lemon juice, and salt. Bring to a boil. Reduce the heat and simmer, covered, for 5 minutes.

2. Spoon the vegetable mixture into a shallow 1½-quart baking dish. Place the fish fillets on top of the vegetables and spoon some of the sauce over the fish.

3. Bake, uncovered, at 400°F for about 15 minutes, or until the fish flakes easily with a fork.

Per serving: 170 calories, 28 g protein, 12 g carbohydrates, 3 g fat, 3 g fiber

STUFFED PEPPERS

6 servings

3	green or red bell peppers	1½	teaspoons cumin
1	can (15 ounces) black beans, rinsed and drained	2	cloves garlic, minced
1	cup corn	¼	cup water
1	cup cooked brown rice	1	ounce low-fat Cheddar cheese, grated
½	cup finely chopped onions	1	ounce jalapeño Jack cheese, grated

1. Preheat the oven to 350°F. Coat a 13" × 9" pan with cooking spray.

2. Cut the peppers in half lengthwise and remove the seeds.

3. In a large bowl, combine the beans, corn, rice, onions, cumin, garlic, and water.

4. Fill each pepper half with the bean mixture and place in the pan. Pour ¼ cup water into the pan. Cover with aluminum foil and bake for 30 minutes.

5. Remove the foil and sprinkle each pepper half with the cheese. Bake, uncovered, for 5 minutes, or until the cheese is melted.

Per serving: 165 calories, 8 g protein, 29 g carbohydrate, 4 g fat, 6 g fiber

SLOPPY JOES

4 servings

1 pound lean ground beef	1 teaspoon mustard
¼ cup chopped onion	¾ cup ketchup
¼ cup chopped green bell pepper	3 teaspoons brown sugar
½ teaspoon garlic powder	Salt and ground black pepper to taste

1. In a medium skillet over medium heat, brown the beef, onion, and bell pepper. Drain off the liquid.

2. Stir in the garlic powder, mustard, ketchup, and brown sugar and mix thoroughly. Reduce the heat and simmer for 30 minutes. Season with the salt and pepper.

Per serving: 350 calories, 28 g protein, 12 g carbohydrates, 16 g fat, 1 g fiber

Variation: Substitute vegetarian crumbles for the ground beef.

ASIAN STEAK

5 servings

1¼	pounds lean flank steak, trimmed of all visible fat
5	cloves garlic, minced
2	tablespoons chopped fresh ginger or 1 teaspoon powdered ginger
⅓	cup vinegar
2	tablespoons soy sauce
½	cup chopped onions
¼	cup water
3	cups fresh spinach, washed and trimmed
1	medium carrot, grated
1	medium tomato, sliced

1. Place the steak in a shallow glass dish.

2. In a food processor, combine the garlic, ginger, vinegar, soy sauce, and ¼ cup of the onions. Blend until smooth.

3. Pour half of the marinade over the steak and turn to coat both sides. Cover and refrigerate for at least 30 minutes. Store the remaining marinade in the refrigerator.

4. Grill or broil the steak for 5 to 7 minutes on each side for medium-rare.

5. Place the remaining marinade in a small saucepan and add the water. Simmer over low heat for 3 to 4 minutes.

6. In a large bowl, toss the remaining onions and the spinach, carrot, and tomato with the warm marinade. Slice the steak into thin strips and serve on the salad.

Per serving: 236 calories, 20 g protein, 6 g carbohydrates, 10 g fat, 2 g fiber

WILD RICE CASSEROLE

6 servings

1	cup brown rice	1	teaspoon garlic powder
½	cup wild rice	1	teaspoon onion powder
1	red bell pepper, chopped	2	tablespoons margarine (no trans fats)
1	green bell pepper, chopped	1	cube vegetable bouillon
1	zucchini, sliced	2	cups hot water
1	carrot, sliced		Salt and ground black pepper to taste
1	rib celery, sliced		

1. Preheat the oven to 350°F.

2. Rinse the rice and pour into a 2-quart baking dish. Add the bell peppers, zucchini, carrot, and celery. Stir in the garlic powder, onion powder, and margarine. Pour the hot water over the bouillon cube to dissolve, then add to the rice mixture and cover.

3. Bake for 30 minutes, then check to see if more water needs to be added. Bake for 15 to 30 minutes longer, or until the rice is cooked. Stir well and season with the salt and pepper.

Per serving: 180 calories, 4 g protein, 31 g carbohydrates, 5 g fat, 4 g fiber

BAKED FRENCH FRIES

6 servings

3 large white or sweet potatoes	1 teaspoon cayenne pepper or ground paprika
1 tablespoon olive oil	Salt and ground black pepper to taste

1. Preheat the oven to 425°F. Coat a baking sheet with cooking spray.

2. Peel the potatoes, if desired. Slice lengthwise into pieces ¼" to ½" thick. In a large bowl, combine the potatoes, oil, and pepper until well coated.

3. Arrange the potatoes in a single layer on the baking sheet. Bake for 45 to 50 minutes, turning occasionally, until crisp. Season with the salt and pepper.

Per serving: 130 calories, 2 g protein, 25 g carbohydrates, 3 g fat, 3 g fiber

WILD RICE APPLE SALAD

6 servings

1 large Granny Smith apple, chopped	¼ cup toasted almonds, sliced (toast raw almonds at 350°F for about 5 minutes)
3 tablespoons fresh lemon juice	
1 cup wild rice, cooked	½ cup orange juice
1½ cups brown rice, cooked	1 tablespoon honey
1 cup chopped celery	1 teaspoon ground coriander
½ cup finely chopped red onions	1 tablespoon olive oil
½ cup raisins	

1. In a large bowl, combine the apple with the lemon juice. Add the rice, celery, onions, raisins, and almonds.

2. In a small bowl, whisk the orange juice, honey, coriander, and oil. Add to the salad mixture and toss to coat.

Per serving: 150 calories, 4 g protein, 27 g carbohydrates, 3 g fat, 3 g fiber

CHICKPEA SALAD WITH RED ONION AND TOMATO

4 servings

1 can (15 ounces) chickpeas, rinsed and drained	½ cup chopped parsley
2 tablespoons chopped red onion	2 tablespoons olive oil
2 cloves garlic, minced	1 tablespoon lemon juice
1 tomato, chopped	Salt and ground black pepper to taste

1. In a large bowl, combine the chickpeas, onion, garlic, tomato, parsley, oil, and lemon juice. Chill for 2 hours before serving. Season with the salt and pepper.

Per serving: 240 calories, 6 g protein, 25 g carbohydrate, 7 g fat, 5 g fiber

ZUCCHINI CASSEROLE

8 servings

1 can (16 ounces) tomato sauce	1 cup cooked whole wheat spaghetti
Salt and ground black pepper to taste	3 medium ribs celery, chopped
1 teaspoon dried oregano	1 medium onion, chopped
½ teaspoon dried basil	1 medium green bell pepper, chopped
2 medium cloves garlic, crushed	8 ounces reduced-fat mozzarella cheese, cut into 18 small slices
4 medium zucchini, sliced	

1. Preheat the oven to 350°F. Lightly coat a 13" × 9" baking dish with cooking spray.

2. In a medium bowl, combine the tomato sauce, salt, pepper, oregano, basil, and garlic.

3. In the baking dish, arrange half the zucchini slices in a single layer. Top with half the spaghetti, celery, onion, and bell pepper. Arrange 9 slices of cheese over the top and spoon half the tomato mixture over the cheese. Repeat the layers.

4. Cover and bake for about 1 hour, or until the vegetables are tender.

Per serving: 135 calories, 10 g protein, 14 g carbohydrate, 5 g fat, 6 g fiber

SWEET CARROT SALAD

8 servings

4	carrots, shredded	2	tablespoons honey
1	apple, peeled, cored, and shredded	¼	cup blanched slivered almonds
1	tablespoon lemon juice		Salt and ground black pepper to taste

1. In a medium bowl, combine the carrots, apple, lemon juice, honey, and almonds. Toss and chill before serving. Season with the salt and pepper.

Per serving: 65 calories, 1 g protein, 11 g carbohydrates, 2 g fat, 2 g fiber

BROCCOLI, ORANGE, AND WATERCRESS SALAD

2 servings

2	medium oranges		Dash of ground black pepper
1	teaspoon vegetable oil	2	cups small broccoli florets
1	teaspoon honey	¼	cup thinly sliced red onion, separated into rings
⅛	teaspoon salt	2	cups trimmed watercress

1. Peel and section the oranges. Squeeze 1 tablespoon juice into a large bowl.

2. Add the oil, honey, salt, and pepper to the orange juice. Stir well and set aside.

3. Steam the broccoli until slightly tender.

4. Add the broccoli, orange sections, onion, and watercress to the orange juice mixture and toss well.

Per serving: 120 calories, 5 g protein, 21 g carbohydrates, 4 g fat, 8 g fiber

ROASTED ASPARAGUS

4 servings

1	pound asparagus, tough ends removed	¼	teaspoon salt
2	teaspoons olive oil	1	clove garlic, minced
1	teaspoon balsamic vinegar		

1. Preheat the oven to 400°F.

2. In a medium bowl, combine the asparagus, oil, vinegar, salt, and garlic until well coated.

3. Arrange the asparagus in a single layer on a baking sheet. Bake for 20 minutes, or until tender.

Per serving: 52 calories, 3 g protein, 0 g carbohydrates, 3 g fat, 2 g fiber

ROASTED VEGETABLES

8 servings

8	zucchini, peeled and chopped	4	tablespoons olive oil
1	eggplant, peeled and chopped	1	teaspoon dried rosemary
8	carrots, chopped	1	teaspoon dried thyme
16	cherry tomatoes	1	teaspoon dried oregano
2	red onions, sliced	2	cloves garlic, minced
1	red bell pepper, sliced		Salt and ground black pepper to taste
1	yellow bell pepper, sliced		

1. Preheat the oven to 400°F.

2. In a large bowl, mix the zucchini, eggplant, carrots, tomatoes, onions, and peppers with the oil, rosemary, thyme, oregano, and garlic.

3. In a large roasting pan, roast the vegetables, uncovered, for 20 minutes, or until the tomatoes split and the edges of the vegetables are slightly crisp. Remove from the oven and stir, then roast for 20 minutes longer. Reduce the heat to 200°F and cook until tender, turning every 20 minutes. Season with the salt and pepper.

Per serving: 165 calories, 5 g protein, 8 g carbohydrates, 7 g fat, 7 g fiber

COLESLAW SALAD

5 servings

2	cups finely shredded green and red cabbage	½	cup low-fat plain yogurt
½	cup finely chopped red or green bell peppers	1	small clove garlic, minced
½	cup finely chopped celery	1	teaspoon fresh lemon juice
¼	cup finely chopped red onions	½	teaspoon ground cumin
¼	cup raisins		

1. In a large bowl, combine the cabbage, peppers, celery, onion, and raisins.

2. In a small bowl, whisk together the yogurt, garlic, lemon juice, and cumin. Add to the salad mixture and toss to coat.

Per serving: 75 calories, 4 g protein, 13 g carbohydrates, 0 g fat, 4 g fiber

GREEN BEANS WITH TOASTED ALMONDS

4 servings

2	cups fresh green beans	1	small onion, finely chopped
1	tablespoon olive oil		Dash of salt
2	tablespoons almonds, sliced	½	teaspoon dried dillweed
1	clove garlic, minced		

1. Steam the green beans in a small amount of water until tender.

2. Heat the oil in a medium skillet. Add the almonds, garlic, and onion and sauté until tender. Add the green beans, salt, and dillweed and cook until heated through.

Per serving: 60 calories, 2 g protein, 6 g carbohydrates, 4 g fat, 3 g fiber

APPLE LADYBUG TREATS

4 servings

2	red apples	1	tablespoon peanut butter
¼	cup raisins	8	thin pretzel sticks

1. Slice the apples in half from top to bottom and scoop out the cores using a knife or melon baller. (If you have an apple corer, core the apples first, then slice.) Place each apple half flat side down on a small plate.

2. Dab peanut butter onto the back of each "ladybug," then stick the raisins into the peanut butter to make spots and eyes. Stick one end of each pretzel stick into a raisin, then press the other end into the apples to make antennae.

Per serving: 118 calories, 2 g protein, 24 g carbohydrates, 3 g fat, 3 g fiber

FRESH HOMEMADE SALSA

4 servings

3	medium tomatoes, chopped	½	cup cilantro, chopped
8	green onions, chopped	1	teaspoon salt
1	green chile pepper, chopped		Juice of 1 lemon

1. In a medium bowl, combine the tomatoes, onions, chile pepper, cilantro, salt, and lemon juice. Enjoy with baked chips or crudités or as a condiment.

Per serving: 20 calories, 0 g protein, 5 g carbohydrates, 0 g fat, 1 g fiber

SPICY BEAN DIP

6 servings

1	cup pinto beans, rinsed and drained	1	clove garlic
1	teaspoon ground cumin	½	small jalapeño pepper, minced and seeds removed

1. In a food processor, combine the beans, cumin, garlic, and peppers. Blend until smooth. Serve with toasted whole wheat pitas, baked chips, or crudités.

Per serving: 80 calories, 5 g protein, 15 g carbohydrates, 0 g fat, 5 g fiber

SPINACH AND ARTICHOKE HEART DIP

8 servings

5	ounces fresh spinach, washed and trimmed	1	cup chopped green onions
2	cloves garlic, minced	2	tablespoons fresh lemon juice
1	can (15 ounces) butter beans, rinsed and drained	1	can (15 ounces) artichoke hearts, chopped

1. Steam the spinach in 2 to 3 tablespoons of water for 2 to 3 minutes, or until wilted. Drain.

2. In a food processor, combine the spinach, garlic, beans, onions, lemon juice, and artichokes. Blend until smooth. Serve with whole wheat pitas or crudités.

Per serving: 50 calories, 4 g protein, 10 g carbohydrates, 0 g fat, 5 g fiber

VEGGIE DIP

4 servings

1 tablespoon minced parsley or 1 teaspoon dried	1 cup low-fat cottage cheese
1 green onion, chopped	2 ounces Boursin or goat cheese
1 teaspoon dried dillweed	

1. In a food processor, combine the parsley, onion, dillweed, cottage cheese, and Boursin. Blend until smooth. Serve with fresh veggies.

Per serving: 90 calories, 10 g protein, 1 g carbohydrates, 2 g fat, 0 g fiber

SPICED PUMPKIN SEEDS

8 servings

1½ tablespoons margarine (no trans fats), melted	2 teaspoons Worcestershire sauce
½ teaspoon salt	2 cups raw whole pumpkin seeds
⅛ teaspoon garlic salt	

1. Preheat the oven to 275°F.

2. In a shallow baking dish, combine the margarine, salt, garlic salt, Worcestershire sauce, and pumpkin seeds. Mix thoroughly and bake for 1 hour, stirring occasionally.

Per serving: 90 calories, 3 g protein, 9 g carbohydrates, 5 g fat, 1 g fiber

FUN FRUIT KEBABS

4 servings

⅓ cup red seedless grapes

⅓ cup green seedless grapes

1 apple, cut into chunks

1 banana, cut into chunks

⅔ cup pineapple chunks

1 cup fat-free yogurt

¼ cup shredded dried coconut

1. Slide the grapes and apple, banana, and pineapple pieces onto 4 skewers, designing your own kebab by using as much or as little of whatever fruit you want. Continue until the skewer is covered almost from end to end.

2. Spread the yogurt onto a large plate and the coconut onto another large plate.

3. Hold each kebab at the ends and roll it in the yogurt so the fruit is covered, then roll it in the coconut.

Per serving: 141 calories, 2 g protein, 28 g carbohydrate, 3 g fat, 3 g fiber

Variation: Try raisins, chopped nuts, or low-fat granola in place of the coconut.

FRUIT SMOOTHIE

1 serving

2 ice cubes

1 cup fat-free or low-fat milk (see note)

⅓ cup low-fat cottage cheese

⅔ cup frozen strawberries

1½ teaspoons sugar

1 teaspoon vanilla extract

2 tablespoons protein powder (optional)

1. In a blender, combine the ice cubes, milk, cottage cheese, strawberries, sugar, and vanilla. Blend for 45 to 60 seconds, or until smooth. Pour into a glass, stir in the protein powder, if using, and serve.

Per serving: 289 calories, 19 g protein, 49 g carbohydrates, 2 g fat, 3 g fiber

Note: Use low-fat milk in smoothies for children age 12 and under. Make the smoothies using fat-free milk for everyone else.

BAKED PEARS

8 servings

8   canned no-sugar-added pear halves, packed in natural juices

½   cup packed brown sugar

1   teaspoon fresh lemon juice

¼   cup unsalted dry-roasted chopped pecans

1. Preheat the oven to 350°F. Drain the pears, reserving the juice. Arrange the pears close together in a baking dish, cut side up.

2. In a small bowl, combine the brown sugar, lemon juice, and pecans. Spoon into the pear halves. Pour the reserved pear juice around the pears to cover the bottom of the dish.

3. Bake for 15 to 20 minutes. Serve warm or cover and refrigerate to serve chilled.

Per serving: 103 calories, 0 g protein, 21 g carbohydrate, 3 g fat, 2 g fiber

VANILLA BERRY PARFAITS

2 servings

2   containers (8 ounces each) low-fat vanilla yogurt

1   package (10 ounces) frozen or fresh mixed berries

2   tablespoons crushed graham crackers

⅛   teaspoon ground nutmeg

1. Cover the bottoms of 2 small glasses with a layer of yogurt, then with a layer of berries. Repeat the layering until both glasses are full, ending with a fruit layer. Sprinkle with the graham crackers and nutmeg.

Per serving: 350 calories, 14 g protein, 65 g carbohydrates, 2 g fat, 3 g fiber

CREAMY RICE PUDDING

6 servings

4	cups fat-free milk	2	eggs, lightly beaten
¼	cup sugar	⅛	teaspoon salt
½	cup raisins	1	teaspoon vanilla extract
½	cup long-grain white or brown rice		Ground cinnamon to taste

1. In a large saucepan over medium-low heat, combine the milk, sugar, raisins, and rice. Simmer, covered, for 30 minutes, or until the rice is tender (45 minutes for brown rice), stirring frequently. Remove from the heat and let stand for 10 minutes.

2. In a small bowl, combine the eggs, salt, and vanilla. Gradually add 1 to 2 cups of the rice mixture to the egg mixture to prevent the eggs from curdling. Stir the egg mixture into the rest of the rice mixture, then return the pot to low heat and cook, stirring constantly, for 2 minutes. Pour into a 13" × 9" baking dish and cover with plastic wrap, folding back the corners to allow the steam to escape.

3. When the pudding has cooled to room temperature, remove the plastic wrap and sprinkle with the cinnamon.

Per serving: 225 calories, 8 g protein, 30 g carbohydrates, 2.5 g fat, 2 g fiber

YUMMY FRUIT SALAD

6 servings

1	can (15 ounces) pineapple chunks with juice	1	banana, sliced
1	apple, peeled, cored, and chopped	1	cup seedless green grapes, halved
1	orange, peeled, chopped, and juice reserved		

1. In a large bowl, toss together the pineapple, apple, orange, banana, and grapes. Add the juice from the pineapple and orange and chill.

Per serving: 106 calories, 1 g protein, 22 g carbohydrates, 0 g fat, 3 g fiber

Variation: Experiment with other fruits, such as kiwifruit, mango, and papaya. You can also add a sprinkling of grated coconut or chopped nuts for a crunchy texture.

APPENDIX B

Michael's Favorite Ways to Get Families Moving

Aerobics—Improves cardiovascular capacity, strengthens the heart, and is great for weight loss. Children 12 and under will get aerobic benefits from their normal activities of running, jumping, and playing sports. Teens and adults can walk, hike, bike, take aerobics classes, use cardiovascular equipment, or play sports.

Badminton—Improves hand-eye coordination, agility, and balance. Badminton is for all ages and is one of my favorite sports for the entire family. Badminton kits are relatively inexpensive, and you can play on just a small piece of your lawn at home or in a park.

Baseball or softball—Improves hand-eye coordination and leg and core strength. This game is great for the entire family and can be played as a simple game of catch, at a batting cage, or as an organized sport.

Basketball—Improves cardiovascular conditioning, hip and leg muscles, and overall athleticism. This is my favorite activity and is great for everyone in the family. If you are old enough to walk and hold a ball in your hands, you can start to play basketball and have fun with shooting, dribbling, and jumping contests.

Biking—Develops leg and hip muscles, core balance, and cardiovascular capacity. Biking is certainly a family activity. You and your family can bike for sport, leisure, or even as transportation. Great for all ages from toddlers on tricycles to adults on mountain bikes.

Bowling—Improves balance, agility, and hand-eye coordination. Millions of Americans bowl regularly for fun and for a night out of the house. Playing on a team with coworkers or friends from the neighborhood can be a great social event while you're getting an activity in. A good source of fun for people age 7 and older.

Boxing—Improves muscle tone, coordination, overall strength, and core development for ages 13 and up. Boxing is one of the toughest workouts, but it is one of the best. It's good for overall body conditioning, weight loss, and self-defense. Always have proper instruction.

Calisthenics—Improves balance, coordination, muscle tone, and strength and is good for weight loss. Calisthenics are "old school," but many exercises are still used today because they work to tone your muscles and get your heart rate up. Jumping rope and doing jumping jacks, pushups, crunches, and back extensions all fall into this category and are especially good for children and teens.

Canoeing—Improves muscle strength and tones arms, shoulders, back, and core. A great outdoor activity for teens and adults. Anytime you can get exercise in the great outdoors, do it. Swimming lessons and life preservers are a must. Okay for most ages with proper adult supervision; I recommend it for those age 7 and older.

Cross-country skiing—Tones the whole body, improves muscle endurance, and enhances cardio, with a focus on arms, legs, and core. This sport and leisure activity is very challenging due to the cold weather and the snowy and sometimes icy surface, and because so many muscles are used at once. Your cardiovascular system is also challenged by the uneven terrain. Proper instruction is a must. Great for all ages; I recommend it for those age 5 and older.

Dancing—Improves cardiovascular capacity, agility, coordination, and balance. John Travolta, step aside! Dancing is one of the best aerobic activities that people of all ages can do. It's perfect as a fun activity indoors or out and lends itself to great socializing.

Dodgeball—Improves athleticism, hand-eye coordination, and cardiovascular capacity. Although it's not played as much today as in years gone by, dodgeball is still a fun activity with a lot of excitement. Play one on one or with two, three, or four players per team. Make sure you use a soft ball and never aim at anyone's head. Fun for all ages.

Downhill skiing—Improves cardiovascular capacity, agility, coordination, balance, and muscle endurance, with a focus on legs and core. Millions across the world practice this Olympic sport and leisure activity. It's fun, challenging, and great exercise for all. Lessons and instruction are highly recommended. Great for all ages with proper instruction. Children belong on slopes designed just for them.

Football—Improves overall muscle endurance as well as cardiovascular capacity. Builds strength, with a focus on legs and core. A widely popular sport and activity, football can be as simple as catch between two people or as complex as a game among 22 players. Organized or not, a game of touch football can be lots of fun. A great form of exercise for any age.

Golf—Improves hand-eye coordination, core strength, and rotation. We all love to play it, but it's just so darn frustrating at times. A game of golf, 9 or 18 holes, is a game of challenge, skill, and coordination. Fun for all ages.

Gymnastics—Improves total-body strength, coordination, agility, and athleticism. This Olympic sport is not always available to everyone, but it is growing in popularity, and many school systems offer it. Ideal for young children and teens, gymnastics can develop the human body to be extremely agile and strong. It's not for everyone, but possibly your child can give it a try by joining an introductory class through school or a private organization.

Hiking—Improves leg muscles and stabilizers at the ankles and knees and strengthens core and cardiovascular capacity. Hiking is great for everyone and is an excellent way to help children begin to be active as well as have fun outdoors with nature. Try trails in your neighborhood, or go crazy and take a family hiking vacation—let's say the Grand Canyon!

Horseback riding—Develops leg and upper-body muscles, with a focus on the core. I love horses because of their beauty and musculature. Horseback riding is a great hobby for kids on ponies or teens and adults on horses. When sitting properly in a saddle, you must use hundreds of muscles in your legs, core, and shoulders. If you have never sat atop a horse, you must try it. It's a total rush and a good form of exercise. Try a lesson or two! Best for ages 7 and above with proper instruction.

Ice hockey or roller hockey—Develops agility, balance, and muscle endurance in the legs, hips, core, and upper body as well as overall strength. Also builds great cardiovascular capacity. I played roller hockey when I was 11 to 15 years old, and it kept me fit and healthy.

It even improved my jumping and running skills in basketball. I recommend it for all children and teens. Adults can also enjoy this activity. Always have proper instruction and protective gear. Take some lessons, join your school team, or play in an after-work league.

Ice skating—Develops agility, balance, and muscle endurance in the legs, hips, core, and upper body. Also builds great cardiovascular capacity. Like any other type of skating, ice skating is a great overall body-conditioning activity. The younger you start, the better you will be at it. Try some lessons, join a skating team, or visit a community rink for a weekend get-together with friends. Great for all ages, but have younger kids try lessons.

Inline skating—Develops agility, balance, and muscle endurance in the legs, hips, core, and upper body as well as overall strength. Also builds great cardiovascular capacity. What a great way to get fit, feel strong, and be outdoors while doing it! Always use protective gear regardless of your experience level. Try a family or individual skate day in an empty parking lot or a designated path along a boardwalk, or commute to school or work. A fun activity for all ages, but I strongly recommend lessons.

Jumping rope—Develops calves and leg muscle strength and endurance as well as coordination and tremendous cardiovascular capacity. Boxers are in such great shape because they jump rope. Jumping rope is the ultimate cardiovascular and conditioning activity. Whether "Double Dutch" or short 1- to 2-minute intervals, I highly recommend it to any and all capable family members. It can be tough on the knees, so check with your physician first. Try to jump rope as intervals during your workouts or as part of a boxing routine.

Karate—Improves balance, coordination, and agility as well as muscle tone and strength. Karate, as well as many other martial arts, is a great activity that is fun and healthy for all family members. I especially like the discipline that is taught with karate and other martial arts; it can be very helpful for maintaining a healthy lifestyle and help with a child's confidence and self-esteem. Try some lessons at a local school or dojo. All age groups in your family can participate for exercise and self-defense.

Kayaking—Improves upper-body tone and strength in arms, shoulders, back, and core. Similar to canoeing or being on a crew team, kayaking requires constant repetition, using the same muscles over and over again. It can be done in calm water or whitewater streams. One-person and two-person kayaks are available. Swimming lessons and life preservers are a must. Great for an individual day trip with family. Best for ages 13 and up.

Kickball—Improves agility, coordination, balance, and athleticism. For hundreds of years, kids all over the world have been kicking balls around in the street or in their yards. You just need a ball to have some fun and get some exercise. Great for all ages.

Pilates—Improves muscle tone, strength, and flexibility, with a focus on the core. Pilates has been around for 50 years but has only recently come to mainstream America. It's a great form of exercise for teens and adults that focuses on flexibility of the entire body and strengthens the core, which I really like. Classes and instruction are easy to find in local health clubs. Try a few lessons, and you will soon feel the benefits. Ages 13 and older.

Rock wall climbing—Develops hand grip and all upper-body muscles as well as core and legs. Also increases cardiovascular capacity. Truly one of the most challenging and exciting activities I have ever tried. Climbing on a rock wall at a health club is the safest and best way for exercisers to work on technique for outdoor climbs. Try climbing on a weekend with the whole family; you'll love it. Appropriate for ages 7 and up. Be sure to have proper instruction and follow safety guidelines.

Running or jogging—Improves speed and strength of leg and core muscles and increases cardiovascular capacity. Other than athletic clothing and footwear, no equipment is needed to get a great workout anywhere in the world; you can even jog or run around the block or your yard, if it's big enough! Proper running shoes are a must to help avoid shinsplints. Always try to run or jog on a surface or terrain that is soft and kind to your knees and hips, such as dirt, sand, or grass. Great for all ages.

Skateboarding—Improves balance, agility, and coordination and helps develop the core. Although I never really got into skateboarding as a kid, everyone I see doing it seems to be having fun. If you do it for long periods of time, you can burn lots of calories. Kids and teens can try it, but stay off the handrails. Wear helmets and elbow and knee pads as well.

Soccer—Improves athleticism, speed, quickness, and leg and core strength as well as overall conditioning and cardiovascular capacity. The most popular sport in the world, soccer is fun, fast, and a great workout for everyone. It's my Week 1 Fit Family Activity recommendation because it's great for anytime. Try joining a school team or soccer club or play in a weekend league. Fun for any age.

Stairclimbing—Improves cardiovascular capacity, builds a strong heart, and conditions your overall body, with an emphasis on the leg muscles. Before there were steppers and stairclimbers, there were just steps in a staircase. Walking or running steps is one of the toughest and most challenging workouts you'll ever take on. Even today, athletes use steps in a stadium to work out. The late, great Walter Payton, Chicago Bears running back, made them famous as part of his off-season routine. Be sure you are advanced before taking on long flights of stairs and high elevations. Try 10 to 12 steps at a time and rest, or do one or two flights at work instead of taking the elevator. Best for those age 13 and older.

Strength training—Develops tone, strength, and power of every single muscle in your body as well as strengthening the heart. As you read in Week 1, I recommend strength training for everyone. Stay consistent with your circuits and intervals and work out as a family whenever you can. Try some personal training sessions to learn new exercises.

Swimming—Improves cardiovascular capacity, muscle flexibility, range of motion of joints, and calorie expenditure. Swimming laps is the most efficient calorie-burning activity we know of because it continuously uses every muscle in your body. It's also great for rehabilitating muscle injuries as well as joint function. Great for kids to learn at an early age.

Tai chi—Improves muscle flexibility, burns calories, improves range of motion, and is mentally and physically soothing. Tai chi is an ancient Chinese art form that is practiced today by millions of people worldwide. It's best known for its slow, deliberate body movements that follow a calming and soothing pattern. It is ideal for individuals who have injuries, loss of strength in muscles, or poor range of motion in joints. It's perfect for adults and seniors who want a low-impact form of exercise, and it can improve a child's agility and coordination. Try taking a class at your local YMCA or community center.

Tennis—Develops lower-body and core muscle strength and tone as well as improving agility, coordination, hand-eye coordination, and speed. Try some lessons for you and the kids, or go to your local park district and have a family game to see who can serve like the pros! Great for all ages once you're strong enough to swing a racket.

Ultimate Frisbee—Improves athleticism, core rotation, coordination, and cardiovascular capacity. Ultimate Frisbee is football with a Frisbee. It is a great deal of fun and can provide nonstop action when played with teams of four, six, and eight people. You just need a Frisbee and an open field. Try a game with your family and friends in the yard, at the beach, or on your next picnic. Okay for ages 7 and up.

Volleyball—Improves athleticism, agility, coordination, overall body conditioning, cardio-vascular capacity, and leg and core power. This is a fantastic sport and activity for everyone. Children under 12 might have some difficulty at first, but growing in height and strength will help. You will condition your body from head to toe by moving in so many directions—and burn excess calories at the same time. Playing in the sand is even more challenging, which will increase your calorie expenditure.

Walking—Improves cardiovascular capacity, strengthens the heart, helps weight loss, tones legs, relieves back pain, improves posture, and helps with circulation. Walking is the perfect activity for everyone. It's the first thing we learn to do as children. The least we should always do is go for a walk. Try intervals of walking on the treadmill at a very steep incline—it'll get your heart rate going!

Water skiing—Improves cardiovascular capacity; overall body conditioning; and leg, hip, core, and upper-body strength. This is one of my favorite activities. Your arms, core, hip, and leg muscles are constantly engaged as you are challenged by an ever-changing surface. Swimming lessons and life vests are a must. Try some lessons or go out on a friend's boat for an afternoon. Best for ages 7 and up.

Wrestling—Develops cardiovascular capacity; builds a strong heart, upper body, core, and lower body; and improves overall body conditioning and toning. Once thought of as only a man's sport, wrestling is now an activity and sport for women. This is an extremely advanced and challenging activity for boys and girls due to the physical and dietary demands. Check with your doctor before entering your child or teen in a wrestling program.

Yoga—Improves overall flexibility and cardiovascular capacity and develops upper-body, core, and lower-body strength as well as balance and agility. The practice of yoga is thousands of years old and is experiencing renewed interest worldwide. Yoga is an advanced flexibility format that incorporates strength movements and a cardiovascular base by warming the body from within. I try to practice weekly because I like the combination with my strength-training circuit routines. It's great for all age groups, but only according to fitness levels. Try a class or two, starting with a beginner or Hatha class if yoga is new to you.

Index